LET'S STOP THE #1 KILLER OF AMERICANS TODAY

A Natural Approach To Preventing
& Reversing Heart Disease

BY

HARRY A. ELWARDT , N.D., PH.D.

Bloomington, IN

authorHOUSE
Milton Keynes, UK

AuthorHouse™
1663 Liberty Drive, Suite 200
Bloomington, IN 47403
www.authorhouse.com
Phone: 1-800-839-8640

AuthorHouse™ UK Ltd.
500 Avebury Boulevard
Central Milton Keynes, MK9 2BE
www.authorhouse.co.uk
Phone: 08001974150

This book is a work of non-fiction. Unless otherwise noted, the author and the publisher make no explicit guarantees as to the accuracy of the information contained in this book and in some cases, names of people and places have been altered to protect their privacy.

First published by AuthorHouse 3/23/2006

ISBN: 1-4259-2321-6 (sc)

Library of Congress Control Number: 2006902206

Printed in the United States of America
Bloomington, Indiana

This book is printed on acid-free paper.

CONTENTS

INTRODUCTION
  The Horrible Truth Be Known..vii

CHAPTER ONE
  Heart Disease Defined 1

CHAPTER TWO
  How Blood Pressure & Diabetes Affect The Heart....................37

CHAPTER THREE
  Causes of Heart Disease 57

CHAPTER FOUR
  Available Tests To Measure Heart Disease Risk.........................73

CHAPTER FIVE
  Conventional Medicine's Answer...95

CHAPTER SIX
  Natural Remedies That Work...123

CONCLUSION 171

REFERENCES 175

INTRODUCTION
The Horrible Truth Be Known

Heart disease is our nation's #1 killer. It has been our #1 cause of death among the American people for the past 80 years. It is a staggering financial burden with estimates as high as 2 billion dollars a day. It is estimated that 1,100,000 new or recurrent heart attacks occur each year in America. Half of all Americans who die this year will die from a heart attack. To better place this disease in perspective, every 20 seconds a person in the United Sates has a heart attack, and every 60 seconds a person will die from one. Often times the very first symptom is the last…a fatal heart attack. That means there is a killer running rampant in the United States who is responsible for the deaths of 2,600 Americans everyday. This is almost the equivalent of the two World Trade Center buildings collapsing each and everyday of the year. And yet more time, money and media exposure is spent securing our country's security from terrorists than securing our protection from this silent killer.

On the death certificate, the doctor might call it "natural causes". Yet, dying of clogged arteries is no more "natural" than being run over by an 18-wheeler! **You can avoid it!** And assuming you survive a heart attack, you are usually so scared that you agree to whatever the cardiologist recommends, anything from an angiogram to bypass surgery. Those with advanced heart disease are told bypass surgery is the only option. What they are not told is that **you can prevent heart disease**, even if you are at high risk; that **you can reverse heart disease**, even if you have had a heart attack; and that **you don't need powerful prescription drugs or surgery** to accomplish this.

The information contained in this book is to help you get a better understanding of this #1 killer of Americans and to guide you into a path of natural healing and prevention. *"We the People"* have been duped into believing lies in the name of big profit. It's time to **Wake Up America** and take control of our own health! You've heard the saying: "You can pay me now or you can pay me later!" Well in this case you will pay later with more than just your finances; you will also pay with unnecessary pain and suffering, and maybe even your life.

I'm not much of a statistics guy, but it's true: every other person you know is likely to die of heart disease. However, my fellow American, you don't have to worry about being a statistic, because I have a battle plan, and the first rule of engagement is: **"In order to defeat your enemy, you must first know your enemy."** So let us begin by learning as much as we can about this cold and merciless killer.

CHAPTER ONE
Heart Disease Defined

Since 1900, heart disease has been the #1 killer in the United States every year except 1918, the year of the great influenza epidemic. Heart disease is directly responsible for over 40% of all health-related deaths in this country and is either the primary or a major contributing factor in 70% of all health-related deaths. In fact, every 29 seconds someone in America dies as a result of heart disease. That is equivalent to a fully loaded 747 aircraft falling out of the sky each and everyday. And here's a sobering statistic: 50% of the time, the first symptom of heart disease is cardiac arrest. Without any prior warning, half of the people who have heart disease die without ever knowing they had it.

And heart disease is not just a man killer. **More than 500,000 women die in the U.S. each year of heart disease,** making it, not breast cancer (40,000 deaths annually), women's #1 killer. Yet ask any American woman what disease they fear most, and the vast majority will answer without hesitation: breast cancer.

Let's begin by looking inside the heart

Your heart is an amazing organ. It continuously pumps oxygen and nutrient-rich blood throughout your body to sustain life. From the moment it begins beating, until the moment it stops, the human heart works tirelessly. In an average lifetime, the heart beats more than two and a half billion times, without ever pausing to rest. Like a pumping machine, the heart provides the power needed for life. This fist-sized powerhouse beats (expands and contracts) 100,000 times per day, pumping five to six quarts of blood each minute, or about 2000 gallons every 24 hours. That is equivelant to 36.6 fifty-five barrel drums each and everyday!

For seventy, eighty or more years, your heart beats slightly more than once each second, contracting and propelling about three ounces per beat of freshly oxygenated blood into your aorta, the large blood vessel attached to your heart muscle. The blood then winds its way into your body's vascular system, including the coronary arteries, which embrace the heart and send the blood further on in its travels.

Blood is essential. In addition to carrying fresh oxygen from the lungs and nutrients to your body's tissues, it also takes the body's waste products, including carbon dioxide, away from the tissues. This is necessary to sustain life and promote the health of all the body's tissues.

This vast system of blood vessels (arteries, veins and capillaries) is over 100,000 miles long. That is long enough to go around the world more than twice; and get this, your blood makes a complete voyage through the body about once a minute. Wow! **We are fearfully and wonderfully made!**

Blood flows continuously through your body's blood vessels. Your heart is the pump that makes it all possible. We never give it a thought until we feel it flutter, and definitely take it for granted right up until it stops.

Heart disease is a term used to describe a disease of the blood vessels or coronary arteries, which supply the heart muscle with vital oxygen and nutrients. When you think of heart disease, usually people think of coronay heart disease (narrowing of the arteries leading to the heart), but coronary heart disease is just one form of a much broader disease known as cardiovascular disease. Let's investigate and get a better understanding of the many different forms of cardiovascular disease.

FORMS OF CARDIOVASCULAR DISEASE

Current estimates are that over 72 million individuals in this country have at least one type of cardiovascular disease. "Cardio" means heart and "vascular" means blood vessels. That is roughly one-third of the adult population; in fact, it's been said that each of us falls into one of two categories: 1) You have cardiovascular problems and know about them or 2) You have cardiovascular problems and do not know about them. Of those that have cardiovascular disease, over 52 million people have high blood pressure, 12.5 million have heart disease, 4.5 million have experienced a stroke, 1 million have congenital cardiovascular defects, and almost 500,000 suffer from congestive heart failure.

Cardiovascular disease is not just a problem for older people. New research also indicates that 60% of 5 to 10 year olds have at least one of the risk factors for cardiovascular disease including high blood pressure, high cholesterol or elevated blood sugar. Few people realize that vascular problems can begin at a very young age and we are now witnessing more and more young people are falling victim to heart problems. During the Vietnam War, autopsies performed on 18 and 19 year old soldiers showed that some of these boys had arteries equivalent to 70 year-old men in the late stages of cardiovascular disease.

So when you hear the word "cardiovascular disease," do not automatically think of heart attack. Heart attacks are just one type of cardiovascular disease. Here is a little more background on the most common forms, including heart attacks and stroke.

ATHEROSCLEROSIS

This disease comes from the Greek words: *athero* meaning gruel or paste and *sclerosis* meaning hardness. Sometimes referred to as the **"silent killer"**, atherosclerosis and cardiovascular disease can progress for years undetected by an individual who may have, or be at great risk from the disease.

Atherosclerosis occurs when the arteries become clogged and narrowed, restricting blood flow to the heart. Without adequate blood, the heart becomes starved of oxygen and vital nutrients it needs to work properly.

This is a slow, progressive disease that may start in childhood. Generally few symptoms arise within the early stages and in some cases even the later stages of the disease. An elevated or high blood pressure for an individual may be an indication of disease presence; however, blood pressure is associated with many other factors such as being overweight, lack of exercise, higher blood sugar, and cholesterol.

This disease progresses rapidly in the 30's and early 40's of some people, while in others it does not become threatening until later in life. Atheroscerosis involves the slow build-up of deposits of fatty substances, cholesterol, body cellular waste products, calcium, and fibrin (a clotting material in the blood) in the inside lining of an artery.

In Chapter 6 we will look at the incredible medical science showing how arginine derived nitric oxide can prevent and reverse atherosclerosis.

CORONARY ARTERY DISEASE (CAD)

Coronary artery disease, also called coronary heart disease, or simply, heart disease, affects more than 13 million Americans and about 515,000 will die this year from the disease. This is the most common form of heart disease and is caused by atherosclerosis, which is hardening (also referred to as arteriosclerosis) and thickening of the coronary arteries.

Coronary artery disease is caused by the buildup that results from atheroscerosis, called plaque, which may partially or totally block the blood's flow through one or all of the coronary arteries, restricting blood flow to the heart. Plaque can grow large enough to significantly reduce blood flow. Most damage occurs when arteries become fragile and rupture. Plaque that ruptures cause blood clots (thrombus) to form that can block blood flow or break off and travel to another part of the body. In either case, without adequate blood, the heart becomes starved of oxygen and vital nutrients it needs to work properly and a heart attack or stroke may result.

Before your teen years, fat starts to deposit in the blood vessel walls. As you get older, the fat builds up. This causes injury to your blood vessel walls. In an attempt to heal itself, the cells release chemicals that make the walls sticky.

Then, other substances such as inflammatory cells, proteins and calcium that travel in your bloodstream start sticking to the vessel walls. The fat and other substances combine to form a material called plaque. The plaque builds up and narrows the artery (atherosclerosis).

Over time, the inside of the arteries develop plaques of different sizes. Many of the plaque deposits are hard on the outside and soft and mushy on the inside. The hard surface can crack or tear, exposing the soft, fatty inside. When this happens, platelets (disc-shaped particles in the blood that aid clotting) come to the area, and blood clots form around the plaque. This causes the artery to narrow even more. Sometimes, the blood clot breaks apart by itself, and blood supply is restored.

Over time a narrowed coronary artery may develop new blood vessels that go around the blockage to get blood to the heart. However, during times of increased exertion or stress, the new arteries may not be able to supply enough oxygen-rich blood to the heart muscle.

In other cases, the blood clot may totally block the blood supply to the heart muscle, causing what is called an acute coronary syndrome. This is actually a name given to three serious conditions: unstable angina (warning sign indicating a possible upcoming heart attack), NSTEMI (a type of heart attack or myocardial infarction that does not cause typical changes on an electrocardiogram; however, chemical markers in the blood indicate that damage has occurred to the heart muscle), and STEMI (a type of heart attack or myocardio infarction, which is caused by a prolonged period of blocked blood supply and does cause typical changes on an electrocardiogram as well as chemical markers in the blood).

Some people have symptoms that tell them that they may soon develop an acute coronary syndrome, others may have no symptoms until something happens, and still others have no symptoms of the acute coronary syndrome at all.

When plaque and fatty matter narrow the inside of an artery to a point where it cannot supply enough oxygen-rich blood to meet your organ's needs, cramping of the muscle occurs. This is called ischemia.

Ischemia of the heart can be compared to a cramp in the leg. When someone exercises for a very long time, the muscles in the legs cramp up because they are starved for oxygen and nutrients. Your heart, also a muscle, needs oxygen and nutrients to keep working. If its blood supply is inadequate to meet the heart muscle's needs, ischemia occurs, and you may feel chest pain or other symptoms.

Ischemia is most likely to occur when the heart demands extra oxygen. This is most common during: exertion (activity), eating, excitement or stress, or exposure to cold.

Coronary artery disease can progress to a point where ischemia occurs even at rest. When ischemia is relieved in a short period of time (less than 10 minutes) with rest or medications, you may be told you have "stable coronary artery disease" or "stable angina."

The most common symptom of coronary artery disease is angina or "angina pectoris," also known as chest pain. Angina can be described as a discomfort, heaviness, pressure, aching, burning, fullness, squeezing or painful feeling. Sometimes, it can be mistaken for indigestion.

Some common symptoms of a coronary artery disease are:

- Angina
- Shortness of breath

- Palpitations (irregular heart beats, skipped beats or a "flip-flop" feeling in your chest)
- A faster heartbeat
- Weakness or dizziness
- Nausea
- Sweating

If you have any of these symptoms, seek medical attention immediately!

In Chapter 6 we will look at the medical science showing how arginine derived nitric oxide can prevent and reverse coronary artery disease.

SUDDEN CARDIAC DEATH (SCD)

This cardiac event accounts for 300,000 deaths each year and is not a "heart attack" caused by clogged arteries. More people die from SCD than AIDS, breast cancer and lung cancer combined.

SCD stems from an electrical problem in which the cardiac conduction system, that generates impulses regulating the heart, suddenly outputs rapid or chaotic electrical impulses, or both. The heart ceases its rhythmic contractions, the brain is starved of oxygen and the victim looses consciousness within seconds. It kills its victims within minutes; 95% die before reaching the hospital, 70% die at home and every 60 seconds the survival rate is reduced by 10%. And get this, 100,000 of those who succumb to this quick and ruthless killer are athletes, in who appear to be in excellent physical condition; in fact 45,000 are basketball players. SCD cares little about multi-million dollar contracts! Defibrillators, which are used to shock the heart back into beating, are becoming as commonplace as fire extinguishers. You can now even purchase one for your own personal protection.

SCD starts with an irregular heartbeat, which is also referred to as an **arrhythmia**. Heart rates can also be irregular. A normal heart rate is 50 to 100 beats per minute. Arrhythmias and abnormal heart rates do not necessarily occur together. Arrhythmias can occur with a normal heart rate, or with heart rates that are slow (called bradyarrhythmias -- less than 60 beats per minute). Arrhythmias can also occur with rapid heart rates (called tachyarrhythmias -- faster than 100 beats per minute). In the United States more than 850,000 people are hospitalized for an arrhythmia each year.

The cause for arrhythmias can be any number of factors including, coronary heart disease, a prior heart attack, changes in your heart muscle, electrolyte imbalances in your blood or something as simple as a lack of vitamin B1, Omega 3-6 or CoQ10 (more about this in Chapter 6).

There are several types of arrhythmias, but let us only look at the ones that are more prevalent in people today:

Ventricular fibrillation. An erratic, disorganized firing of impulses from the ventricles (the lower chambers of the heart). The ventricles quiver and are unable to contract or pump blood to the body. This is a medical emergency that must be treated with cardiopulmonary resuscitation (CPR) and defibrillation as soon as possible. Sudden cardiac death can be caused by ventricular fibrillation. The heart fibrillates (quivers) and stops pumping blood to the body. Although there are other causes of sudden cardiac death, the majority is due to ventricular fibrillation.

Atrial Fibrillation. According to the American Heart Association, one out of every four adults over the age of 40 could develop atrial fibrillation, which is defined as an irregular heartbeat. Approximately 2.2 million people living in the United States have been diagnosed with atrial fibrillation. This condition accounts for almost 15 to 20% of stroke cases and is considered the most common of heart rhythm disorders. It could also lead to a number of negative health repercussions such as an increased risk of stroke, death and an overall reduction in the quality of life.

Atrial fibrillation causes a quivering in the two upper chambers of the heart, known as the atria, as opposed to having it beat effectively. When this happens, blood is unable to pump completely out of these chambers, which could then lead to clotting. The formation of blood clots could then travel from the heart to the brain, which results in an ischemic stroke.

Atrial fibrillation is often a "silent" condition, meaning that some patients do not detect any changes with their heart rhythm and therefore are walking around undiagnosed, oblivious to the fact they have the condition. Researchers from a study of medical histories and electrocardiograms concluded that once a person turned 40 years of age, their average lifetime risk for developing atrial fibrillation was 26% for men and 23% for women. To put these findings into perspective, researchers took the lifetime risk for breast cancer for a 70-year-old woman, which is one in 14, and compared it to that same person's remaining lifetime risk of atrial fibrillation, one in four and stressed the importance of looking into taking a more preventative approach to atrial fibrillation and finding some more effective forms of therapy.

Premature Ventricular Contractions (PVCs). These are among the most common arrhythmias and occur in people with and without heart disease. This is the skipped heartbeat we all occasionally experience. In some people, it can be related to stress, too much caffeine or nicotine, or too much exercise. But sometimes, PVCs can be caused by heart disease or electrolyte imbalance. People who have a lot of PVCs, and/or symptoms associated with them, should be evaluated by a heart doctor. However, in most people, PVCs are usually harmless and rarely need treatment.

Premature Atrial Contractions. These are early, extra beats that originate in the atria (upper chambers of the heart). They are harmless and do not require treatment.

Bradyarrhythmias. These are slow heart rhythms, which may arise from disease in the heart's electrical conduction system. Examples include sinus node dysfunction and heart block and are often treated with a pacemaker.

Ventricular Tachycardia (V-tach). A rapid heart rhythm originating from the ventricles (lower chambers) of the heart. The rapid rate prevents the heart from filling adequately with blood; therefore, less blood is able to pump through the body. This can be a serious arrhythmia, especially in people with heart disease, and may be associated with more symptoms. A heart doctor should evaluate this arrhythmia.

Some common symptoms of arrhythmias:

- Palpitations (a feeling that your heart is fluttering, skipping beats, or beating excessively)
- Pounding in your chest
- Dizziness or feeling light headed
- Shortness of breath
- Chest discomfort
- Fainting
- Feeling tired or weak

On the other hand, an arrhythmia can be silent and not cause any symptoms. A doctor can detect an irregular heartbeat during a physical exam by taking your pulse or through an electrocardiogram (ECG).

If you have any of these symptoms, seek medical attention immediately!

Conventional treatment for arrhythmias should begin with some common sense lifestyle changes like stop smoking, limit your intake of alcohol, limit or stop using caffeine (some people are sensitive to caffeine and may notice more symptoms when using caffeine products such as tea, coffee, colas and some over-the-counter medications), stay away from stimulants used in cough and cold medications. Such medications contain ingredients that promote irregular heart rhythms. Read the label and ask your doctor or pharmacist what medication would be best for you.

Next your doctor will try antiarrhythmic drugs (controls heart rate) and/or anticoagulant drugs (reduce blood clots and strokes).

If drugs are not able to control a persistent irregular heart rhythm more invasive procedures may be necessary:

- **Electrical Cardioversion** is an electrical shock delivered to your chest wall (after administering an anesthesia) that synchronizes the heart and allows the normal rhythm to restart.

- **Pacemaker** is a device that sends small electrical impulses to the heart muscle to maintain a suitable heart rate. Pacemakers primarily prevent the heart from beating too slowly. The pacemaker has a pulse generator (which houses the battery and a tiny computer) and leads (wires) that send impulses from the pulse generator to the heart muscle. Newer pacemakers have many sophisticated features that are designed to help manage arrhythmias and optimize heart-rate-related function as much as possible.

- **Implantable Cardioverter-Defribrillator (ICD)** is a sophisticated device used primarily to treat ventricular tachycardia and ventricular fibrillation, two life-threatening heart rhythms. The ICD constantly monitors the heart rhythm. When it detects a very fast, abnormal heart rhythm, it delivers energy to the heart muscle to cause the heart to beat in a normal rhythm again. There are several ways the ICD can be used to restore normal heart rhythm. They include:
  1. **Anti-tachycardia pacing (ATP).** When the heart beats too fast, a series of small electrical impulses may be delivered to the heart muscle to restore a normal heart rate and rhythm.
  2. **Cardioversion.** A low energy shock may be delivered at the same time as the heart beats to restore normal heart rhythm.
  3. **Defibrillation.** When the heart is beating dangerously fast or irregularly, a higher energy shock may be delivered to the heart muscle to restore a normal rhythm.
  4. **Anti-bradycardia pacing.** Many ICDs provide back-up pacing to prevent too slow of a heart rhythm.

- **Catheter Ablation** is a non-surgical procedure performed in a special lab called the electrophysiology (EP) laboratory. During this non-surgical procedure a catheter is inserted into your heart and then a special machine is used to direct energy to the heart muscle. This energy either "disconnects" or "isolates" the pathway of the abnormal rhythm (depending on the type of ablation). It can also be used to disconnect the electrical pathway between the upper chambers (atria) and the lower chambers (ventricles) of the heart. This procedure can also be performed surgically.

- **Heart Surgery** may be needed to correct heart disease that may be causing the arrhythmia. The Maze procedure is a type of surgery used to correct atrial fibrillation. During this procedure, a series (or "maze") of incisions are made in the right and left atria to confine the electrical impulses to defined pathways. Some people may require a pacemaker after this procedure.

In Chapter 6 we will look at natural ways to prevent sudden cardiac death and reverse arrhythmias.

CONGESTIVE HEART FAILURE

The *National Heart, Lung, and Blood Institute (NHLBI)* say an estimated 5 million Americans have congestive heart failure (CHF). And the numbers are on the rise. CHF is a progressive cardiac illness in which the heart cannot pump enough oxygenated blood to meet the body's needs. Failure does not mean that the heart has stopped pumping but rather that it is failing to pump as effectively as it should.

The body tries to compensate for the reduced pumping ability of your heart by: retaining salt and water to increase the amount of blood in your bloodstream, increasing your heart rate, or increasing the size of your heart. An enlarged heart is called cardiomegaly.

Congestive heart failure is caused by diseases or factors that ultimately affect the pumping ability of the heart, specifically the left ventricle chamber of the heart. Among them are aging (your heart muscle stiffens with age), cornary artery disease, heart attack, high blood pressure, diabetes, thyroid problems, myocarditis (infection or inflammation of the heart muscle), congenital heart disease, heart valve disease, or arrhythmias (irregular heart beat).

The *American Heart Association (AHA)* estimates there are over 500,000 new cases of congestive heart failure each year. The annual number of deaths directly related to congestive heart failure is increasing too, and it is the most common diagnosis in hospital patients age 65 years and older. There is no cure for CHF but people do live with the condition. According to *AHA*, managing congestive heart failure involves medications and changes in diet and lifestyle along with treatment for the underlying conditions that caused the congestive heart failure. But I also know of many people with congestive heart failure who are now living normal lives because of supplementing with arginine and other nutritional supplements, but more about these forms of therapy in Chapter 6.

Some common symptoms of congestive heart failure are:

- Shortness of breath from exertion, while lying down or while sleeping
- Weight gain
- Swelling in the feet or ankles
- Fatigue, inability to exercise or decrease in muscle strength
- Abdominal swelling, tenderness and/or pain
- Decrease in appetite
- Increase in urination
- Dry hacking cough, worse when lying down

If you have any of these symptoms, seek medical attention immediately!

In Chapter 6 we will look at natural solutions that will greatly improve the quality of life in someone with congestive heart failure.

HEART VALVE DISEASE

According to the *American Heart Association*, about 5 million Americans are diagnosed with valvular heart disease each year. Heart valve disease occurs when the heart valves do not work the way they should.

Your heart valves lie at the exit of each of your four heart chambers and maintain one-way blood flow through your heart. The four heart valves make sure that blood always flows freely in a forward direction and that there is no backward leakage.

Blood flows from your right and left atria into your ventricles through the open mitral and tricuspid valves. When the ventricles are full, the mitral and tricuspid valves shut. This prevents blood from flowing backward into the atria while the ventricles contract (squeeze).

As the ventricles begin to contract, the pulmonic and aortic valves are forced open and blood is pumped out of the ventricles through the open valves into the pulmonary artery toward the lungs, the aorta, and the body.

When the ventricles finish contracting and begin to relax, the aortic and pulmonic valves snap shut. These valves prevent blood from flowing back into the ventricles.

This pattern is repeated over and over, causing blood to flow continuously to the heart, lungs and body.

Valve disease can develop before birth (congenital) or can be acquired sometime during one's lifetime. Sometimes the cause of valve disease is unknown.

The most common causes of valve disease include:

- **Mitral valve prolapse (MVP)**, which is a very common condition, affecting 1 to 2 percent of the population. MVP causes the leaflets of the mitral valve to flop back into the left atrium during the heart's contraction. MVP also causes the tissues of the valve to become abnormal and stretchy, causing the valve to leak. The condition rarely causes symptoms and usually does not require treatment.

- **Endocarditis** occurs when germs, especially bacteria, enter the bloodstream and attack the heart valves, causing growths and holes in the valves and scarring, which can lead to leaky valves.
- **Rheumatic fever** caused by an untreated bacterial infection, usually strep throat. The initial infection usually occurs in children, but the heart problems associated with the infection may not be seen until 20-40 years later. Thanks to antibiotics the number of infections have been dramatically reduced.
- **Other causes** include coronary artery disease, heart attack, cardiomyopathy (heart muscle disease), syphilis (a sexually transmitted disease), hypertension, aortic aneurysms, and connective tissue diseases. Less common causes of valve disease include tumors, some types of drugs and radiation.

Symptoms do not always relate to the seriousness of your valve disease. You may have no symptoms at all and have severe valve disease, requiring prompt treatment, or you may have severe symptoms, as with mitral valve prolapse, yet tests may show your valve leak is not significant.

Some common symptoms of a heart valve disease are:

- Shortness of breath and/or difficulty catching your breath
- Weakness or dizziness
- Discomfort in your chest (usually with activity or going out in cold air)
- Palpitations (irregular heart beat)
- Swelling of your ankles, feet or abdomen (also called edema)
- Rapid weight gain (2-3 pounds in one day is possible)

CONGENITAL HEART DISEASE

About 500,000 adults in the U.S. have congenital heart disease. This disease is a type of defect or malformation in one or more structures of the heart or blood vessels that occurs before birth.

These defects occur while the fetus is developing in the uterus and affect 8 to 10 out of every 1,000 children. Congenital heart defects may produce symptoms at birth, during childhood or sometimes not until adulthood.

In the majority of people, the cause of congenital heart disease is unknown. However, there are some factors that are associated with an increased chance of getting congenital heart disease. These risk factors include:

- Genetic or chromosomal abnormalities in the child such as Down Syndrome
- Taking certain medications or alcohol or drug abuse during pregnancy
- Maternal viral infection, such as rubella (German measles) in the first trimester of pregnancy

The risk of having a child with congenital heart disease is higher if a parent or a sibling has a congenital heart defect; in fact, the risk increases from 8 in 1000 to 16 in 1000.

The most common congenital heart problems include heart valve defects, heart muscle abnormalties and defects in the walls between the atria and ventricles of the heart.

Congenital heart defects may be diagnosed before birth, right after birth, during childhood or not until adulthood. It is possible to have a defect and no symptoms at all.

Some common symptoms of congenital heart disease in adults are:

- Shortness of breath
- Limited ability to exercise

HEART MUSCLE DISEASE (CARDIOMYOPATHY)

This is a type of progressive heart disease in which the heart is abnormally enlarged, thickened and/or stiffened. As a result, the heart muscle's ability to pump blood is weakened, often causing heart failure and the backup of blood into the lungs or rest of the body. This disease can also cause abnormal heart rhythms.

Usually, the condition begins in the heart's lower chambers (the ventricles), but in severe cases can affect the upper chambers or atria as well.

There are three main types of cardiomyopathy:

- **Dilated cardiomyopathy (DCM)** is a condition in which the heart's ability to pump blood is decreased because the heart's main pumping chamber, the left ventricle, is enlarged and stiff; this causes a decreased ejection fraction (the amount of blood pumped out with each heart beat). In some cases, it prevents the heart from relaxing and filling with blood as it should. Over time, it can affect the other heart chambers as well. DCM can be inherited, but it is primarily caused by a variety of other factors including severe coronary artery disease, alcoholism, thyroid disease, diabetes, viral infections of the heart, heart valve abnormalties and drugs that are toxic and cause damage to the heart.
- **Hypertrophic cardiomyopathy (HCM)** is associated with thickening of the heart muscle, most commonly at the septum between the ventricles, below the aortic valve. This leads to stiffening of the walls of the heart and abnormal aortic and

mitral heart valve function, both of which may impede normal blood flow out of the heart. HCM can run in families, but the condition may also be acquired as a part of aging or high blood pressure. In other instances, the cause is unknown.

- **Restrictive cardiomyopathy (RCM)** is the rarest form of cardiomyopathy. It is a condition in which the walls of the lower chambers of the heart (the ventricles) are abnormally rigid and lack the flexibility to expand as the ventricles fill with blood. The pumping or systolic function of the ventricle may be normal but the diastolic function (the ability of the heart to fill with blood) is abnormal. Therefore, it is harder for the ventricles to fill with blood, and with time, the heart loses the ability to pump blood properly, leading to heart failure. RCM may be caused by chemotherapy or chest exposure to radiation, excess iron in the heart, build-up of abnormal proteins in the heart, or build-up of scar tissue (often for no known reason).

Some common symptoms of heart muscle disease are:

- Chest pain or pressure (occurs usually with exercise or physical activity, but can also occur with rest or after meals)
- Heart failure symptoms (shortness of breath and fatigue)
- Swelling of the lower extremities
- Fatigue (feeling overly tired)
- Weight gain
- Fainting (caused by irregular heart rhythms, abnormal responses of the blood vessels during exercise, or no cause may be found)
- Palpitations (fluttering in the chest due to abnormal heart rhythms)
- Dizziness or lightheadedness
- Sudden death occurs in a small number of patients with HCM
- Nausea, bloating and poor appetite (related to fluid retention) with RCM

PERICARDIAL DISEASE

Also called pericarditis, is inflammation of any of the layers of the pericardium. The pericardium is a thin fibrous membrane sac that surrounds the heart and consists of:

- An inner layer (visceral pericardium) that envelopes the entire heart
- An outer layer (parietal pericardium) comprising the outer fibrous sac
- A middle fluid layer to prevent friction between the parietal pericardium and visceral pericardium

Causes of pericarditis include infections, heart surgery, heart attack, trauma, tumors, cancer, radiation, autoimmune diseases (such as rheumatoid arthritis, lupus, or scleroderma). For some people, no cause can be found.

Pericarditis can be acute (occurring suddenly) or chronic (long-standing).

Some common symptoms of pericardial disease are:

- Low grade fever
- Increased heart rate
- Chest pain. This pain is different from angina (pain caused by coronary artery disease). It may be sharp and located in the center of the chest. The pain may radiate to the neck and occasionally, the arms and back. It is made worse when lying down, coughing or swallowing and relieved by sitting forward.

AORTIC ANEURYSM

An aneurysm is an abnormal bulge in the wall of an artery. Normally, the walls of arteries are thick and muscular, allowing them to withstand a large amount of pressure. Occasionally, however, a weak area develops in the wall of an artery. This allows the pressure within the artery to push outward, creating a bulge or ballooned area called an "aneurysm."

Aneurysms can form in any blood vessel, but they occur most commonly in the aorta (aortic aneurysm). The aorta is the largest artery in the body. It carries blood from the heart to the rest of the body. Aortic aneurysms can occur in two main places:

- Abdominal aortic aneurysms occur in the part of the aorta that passes through the middle to lower abdomen.
- Thoracic aortic aneurysms occur on the aorta as it passes through the chest cavity. These are less common than abdominal aneurysms.

Small aneurysms generally pose no threat. However, aneurysms increase the risk for:

- Atherosclerotic plaque formation at the site of the aneurysm. This causes further weakening of the artery wall.
- A blood clot may form at the site and dislodge, increasing the chance of stroke.
- Increase in the size of the aneurysm, causing it to press on other organs. This may cause pain.
- Aneurysm rupture. Because the artery wall thins at this spot, it is fragile and may burst under stress. The rupture of an aortic aneurysm is a catastrophic, life-threatening event.

Aneurysms may be caused by:

- Atherosclerosis, or hardening of the arteries, which weakens arterial walls
- Hypertension (high blood pressure)
- Local injury to the artery
- Congenital abnormality. A number of conditions, such as Marfan syndrome, are present at birth and can cause weakness of the artery walls.
- Aging

- Syphilis use to be a common cause of thoracic aneurysms, but that is no longer as common

Note: Instead of causing a bulge in a thinned artery wall, aortic aneurysms occasionally occur between layers of the artery itself. This is called a "dissecting aneurysm." Blood starts to flow in the separated artery layers cutting off blood flow in the artery. This condition can rapidly lead to rupture of the artery.

Some common symptoms of aortic aneurysms are:

- Tearing pain in the chest, abdomen and/or middle of the back between the shoulder blades
- Thoracic aneurysms may cause shortness of breath, hoarseness, brassy cough (due to pressure on the lungs and airways) and difficulty swallowing (pressure on the esophagus)
- Rupture of an aneurysm can cause loss of consciousness, stroke, shock or a heart attack

If you have any of these symptoms, seek medical attention immediately!

In Chapter 6 we will explore the medical science, which shows how arginine derived nitric oxide will prevent aneurysms.

MARFAN SYNDROME

This is an inherited disease that affects the connective tissue. Connective tissue is the most abundant tissue in the body and is a vital component to supporting the body's organs. Its primary purpose is to hold the body together and provide a framework for growth and development. It provides the strength and support to tendons, cartilage, heart valves and many other parts of the body, as well as strength and elasticity to the blood vessels.

For people with Marfan syndrome, the chemical makeup of the connective tissue is not normal and as a result is not as strong as it should be. Because connective tissue is found throughout the body, Marfan syndrome can affect many parts, including the bones, eyes, heart and blood vessels, nervous system, skin and lungs.

Marfan syndrome is caused by a defect in the gene that encodes the structure of fibrillin, and the elastic fibers, which are major and essential components of connective tissue that appears to contribute to its strength and elasticity.

In most cases, Marfan syndrome is inherited. The pattern is called "autosomal dominant," meaning it occurs equally in men and women and can be inherited from just one parent with the disorder. People with Marfan syndrome have a 50% chance of passing along the disorder to their children. In rare cases, a new gene defect occurs due to an unknown cause. Marfan syndrome is also referred to as a "variable expression" genetic disorder, since everyone with Marfan syndrome has the same defective gene, but not everyone experiences the same symptoms to the same degree.

Marfan syndrome is present at birth. However, the condition may not be diagnosed until adolescence or young adulthood. It is fairly common, affecting 1 in 5,000 Americans. It is found in people of all races and ethnic backgrounds.

Sometimes Marfan syndrome is so mild, few, if any, symptoms occur. In most cases, the disease progresses with age and symptoms become noticeable as the changes in connective tissue occur.

On the outside, people with Marfan syndrome are often very tall and thin. Their arms, legs, fingers and toes may seem out of proportion, too long for the rest of their body. Their spine may be curved and their breastbone (sternum) may either stick out or be indented inward. Their joints may be weak and easily become dislocated. Often, people with Marfan syndrome have a long, narrow face and the roof of the mouth may be higher than normal, causing the teeth to be crowded. More than half of all people with Marfan syndrome have eye problems.

Internally, many changes occur within the body structures due to the abnormal connective tissue. About 90% of people with Marfan syndrome develop changes in their heart and blood vessels.

Some common symptoms of Marfan syndrome are:

- Enlarged and weakened heart (can progress to heart failure)
- Abnormal heart rhythm (arrhythmia)
- Leaky aortic valve
- Mitral valve prolapse, which may cause shortness of breath, feeling over-tired or palpitations (fluttering in the chest)

HEART ATTACK

More than 1 million Americans have heart attacks each year. A heart attack, or myocardial infarction (MI), is permanent damage to the heart muscle. "Myo" means muscle, "cardial" refers to the heart and "infarction" means death of tissue due to lack of blood supply. The heart muscle requires a constant supply of oxygen-rich blood to nourish it. The coronary arteries provide the heart with this critical blood supply. If you have coronary artery disease, those arteries become narrow and blood cannot flow as well as it should.

When the plaque's hard, outer shell cracks (plaque rupture), platelets (disc-shaped particles in the blood that aid clotting) come to the area, and blood clots form around the plaque. If a blood clot totally blocks the artery, the heart muscle becomes "starved" for oxygen. Within a short time, death of heart muscle cells occur, causing permanent damage. This is called a myocardial infarction (MI), or heart attack.

While it is unusual, a heart attack can also be caused by a spasm of a coronary artery. During coronary spasm, the coronary arteries restrict or spasm on and off, reducing blood supply to the heart muscle (ischemia). It may occur at rest and can even occur in people without significant coronary artery disease.

Each coronary artery supplies blood to a region of heart muscle. The amount of damage to the heart muscle depends on the size of the area supplied by the blocked artery and the time between injury and treatment.

Healing of the heart muscle begins soon after a heart attack and takes about eight weeks. Just like a skin wound, the heart's wound heals and a scar will form in the damaged area. But, the new scar tissue does not contract or pump as well as healthy heart muscle tissue. So, the heart's pumping ability is lessened after a heart attack. The amount of lost pumping ability depends on the size and location of the scar.

In most people, the tip-off that the angina (chest pain) they are experiencing is a warning sign and not indigestion, is that the symptoms come on during physical exertion, mental stress, or eating a heavy meal.

Stable angina is a condition in which a person has angina of the same severity for several months or years. This form of chest pain is triggered by activity, but is relieved after resting for a few minutes or by taking a nitroglycerin pill. People with stable angina can live for years without ever having an actual heart attack.

Unstable angina is a condition in which the angina suddenly becomes much worse. The very first time you have angina is actually called unstable angina. This form of chest pain is more severe, the duration is longer and it will take more rest and/or nitroglycerin to relieve it.

During an actual heart attack, symptoms last 30 minutes or longer and are not relieved by rest or oral medications (medications taken by mouth). If you are experiencing any of the symptoms listed below, **do not** pass it off as indigestion. It is important to act quickly, because 50% of people who have a heart attack die before reaching the hospital.

Some people have a heart attack without having any symptoms (a "silent" myocardial infarction). A silent MI can occur in any person, though it is more common among diabetics.

Some common symptoms of a heart attack are:

- Pain or discomfort, pressure, or squeezing sensation in the center of your chest that lasts for more than a few minutes
- Pain or discomfort that radiates to your shoulders, jaw, neck, throat or arms
- Discomfort in your chest that is accompanied by nausea, vomiting, heartburn, sweating, fainting, or a feeling of light-headedness
- Shortness of breath or extreme weakness
- Rapid or irregular heart beats

If you have any of these symptoms, seek medical attention immediately!

In Chapter 6 of this book we will look at the medical science showing how arginine derived nitric oxide can prevent heart attacks.

HEART ATTACK SURVIVORS ARE AT RISK FOR SUDDEN CARDIAC DEATH (SCD)

According to the *American Heart Association,* many heart attack patients never make a complete recovery. About 50% of the men and women under age 65 who have had a heart attack die within eight years of the precipitating event.

A heart attack can damage your heart and create an area of scar tissue. If large enough, this scar tissue may put you at risk for SCD. The scar can unexpectedly create a fast, dangerous heart rhythm. Without immediate treatment, this condition may be lethal.

SCD can strike without warning. Often, those who experience it felt fine moments before. Knowing that a heart attack puts you at risk is your first step in learning about SCD.

Your doctor can determine your risk by measuring the fraction of blood pumped (ejected) by your heart with each heartbeat. Doctors call this measurement the ejection fraction, or EF. The ejection fraction is measured using a simple and painless heart ultrasound called an echocardiogram, or "echo." An echo can be performed easily in your doctor's office in just a few minutes.

A healthy heart pumps at least one-half of the blood it holds with each beat. But after a heart attack, the damaged heart has a reduced ejection fraction. A level of less than one-third dramatically raises the risk for SCD.

In Chapter 6 of this book we will look at the medical science showing how arginine derived nitric oxide can greatly diminish your chances of having a second heart attack.

CAROTID ARTERY DISEASE

Also called carotid artery stenosis, is the narrowing of the carotid arteries, usually caused by the buildup of fat and cholesterol deposits, called plaque. Like the arteries that supply blood to the heart (the coronary arteries), the carotid arteries can also develop atherosclerosis on the inside of the vessels.

There are two carotid arteries (one on each side of the neck) that supply blood to the brain. The carotid arteries can be felt on each side of the neck, immediately below the angle of the jaw.

The carotid arteries supply blood to the large, front part of the brain, where thinking, speech, personality, sensory and motor functions reside.

Over time, the buildup of fat and cholesterol narrows the carotid arteries, decreasing blood flow to the brain and increasing the risk of a stroke. A stroke is similar to a heart attack. It occurs when brain cells (neurons) are deprived of the oxygen and glucose (a sugar) carried to them by blood. Oxygen and glucose are essential for neurons to function and survive. If the lack of blood flow lasts for more than 3 to

6 hours, the damage is usually permanent. A stroke can occur if the artery becomes extremely narrowed, a piece of plaque breaks off and travels to the smaller arteries of the brain or a blood clot forms and blocks a narrowed artery.

A stroke can occur as a result of other conditions, such as sudden bleeding in the brain (intracerebral hemorrhage), sudden bleeding in the spinal fluid space (subarachnoid hemorrhage), atrial fibrillation, cardiomyopathy or blockage of tiny arteries inside the brain.

Typically, the carotid arteries become diseased a few years later than the coronary arteries. People who have coronary artery disease have an increased risk of developing carotid artery disease.

STROKE

Every fifty-three seconds, someone in the United States has a stroke. A death from a stroke takes place every three minutes. 750,000 Americans suffer a symptomatic stroke each year (expected to double in the next 5 years) and another 22 million suffer a silent stroke.

A stroke, sometimes called a "brain attack," occurs when blood flow to an area in the brain is cut off. The brain cells, deprived of the oxygen and glucose needed to survive, die. If not caught early, permanent brain damage can result.

There are two types of strokes. Hemorrhagic strokes occur when a blood vessel in the brain breaks or ruptures. The result is blood seeping into the brain tissue, causing damage to brain cells. The most common causes of hemorrhagic stroke are high blood pressure and brain aneurysms. An aneurysm is a weakness or thinness in the blood vessel wall.

An ischemic stroke is caused by a blood clot that blocks blood flow to the brain. A blood clot can develop in a narrowed artery that supplies the brain or can travel from the heart (or elsewhere in the body) to an artery that supplies the brain.

Blood clots are usually the result of other problems in the body that affect the normal flow of blood, such as: atherosclerosis (hardening of the arteries), atrial fibrillation (irregular heartbeats), mitral valve prolapse (heart valve problem), endocarditis (infection of the heart valves), patent foramen ovale (congenital heart defect), vasculitis (inflammation of the blood vessels), blood clotting disorders or a heart attack.

Some common symptoms of a stroke or transient ischemic attack (TIA):

- Weakness in an arm, hand, or leg
- Numbness, weakness, or paralysis of the face, arm, or leg, typically on one side of the face or body
- Sudden blindness in one eye
- Vision problems in one or both eyes, such as dimness, blurring, double vision, or loss of vision
- Difficulty talking or confusion
- Difficulty understanding what someone is saying
- Dizziness or loss of balance or coordination
- Trouble walking
- Sudden, severe headache

If you have any of these symptoms, seek medical attention immediately!

In Chapter 6 of this book we will look at the medical science showing that arginine derived nitric oxide can prevent a stroke.

VASCULAR DISEASE

As the heart beats, it pumps blood through a system of blood vessels called the circulatory system. The vessels are elastic tubes that carry blood to every part of the body. Arteries carry blood away from the heart while veins return it.

Vascular disease includes any condition that affects your circulatory system. This ranges from diseases of your arteries, veins and lymph vessels to blood disorders that affect circulation. The following are conditions that fall under the category of vascular disease:

PERIPHERAL ARTERY DISEASE (PAD)

The hardening of the arteries in the leg vessels affects 3 million Americans and is one of the most underdiagnosed diseases of the blood vessels. Like the blood vessels of the heart (coronary arteries), your peripheral arteries (blood vessels outside your heart) also may develop atherosclerosis, the build-up of fat and cholesterol deposits, called plaque, on the inside walls. Over time, the build-up narrows the artery. Eventually the narrowed artery causes less blood to flow and a condition called "ischemia" can occur. Ischemia is inadequate blood flow to the body's tissue. A blockage in the legs can lead to leg pain or cramps with activity (a condition called claudication), changes in skin color, sores or ulcers and feeling tired in the legs. People often attribute their leg discomfort to the aches and pains of growing old. However, this can lead to a total loss of circulation, which can then lead to gangrene and critical limb ischemia. 750,000 Americans have critical limb ischemia, resulting in 200,000 amputations each year. Of those that can get a balloon, stent or bypass, 30% fail within a year and 40% die within 4 years due to a heart attack or stroke.

RENAL ARTERY DISEASE

This disease is most commonly caused by atherosclerosis of the renal (kidney) arteries. It occurs in people with generalized vascular disease. Less often, renal artery disease can be caused by a congenital (present at birth) abnormal development of the tissue that makes up the renal arteries. This type of renal artery disease occurs in younger age groups. A blockage in the renal arteries (arteries supplying the kidneys) can cause renal artery disease (stenosis). The symptoms include uncontrolled hypertension (high blood pressure), heart failure and abnormal kidney function.

RAYNAUD'S DISEASE

Also called Raynaud's Syndrome or Raynaud's Phenomenon, consists of spasms of the small arteries of the fingers and sometimes the toes, brought on by exposure to cold or excitement. Certain occupational exposures bring on Raynaud's. The episodes produce temporary lack of blood supply to the area, causing the skin to appear white or bluish and cold or numb. In some cases, the symptoms of Raynaud's may be related to underlying diseases (i.e., lupus, rheumatoid arthritis, scleroderma).

BUEGER'S DISEASE

This disease most commonly affects the small and medium sized arteries, veins and nerves. Although the cause is unknown, there is a strong association with tobacco use or exposure. The arteries of the arms and legs become narrowed or blocked, causing lack of blood supply (ischemia) to the fingers, hands, toes and feet. Pain occurs in the arms, hands and, more frequently, the legs and feet, even when at rest. With severe blockages, the tissue may die (gangrene), requiring amputation of the fingers and toes. Superficial vein inflammation and symptoms of Raynaud's occur commonly in patients with Buerger's Disease.

PERIPHERAL VENOUS DISEASE

Veins are flexible, hollow tubes with flaps inside called valves. When your muscles contract, the valves open and blood moves through the veins. When your muscles relax, the valves close, keeping blood flowing in one direction through the veins. If the valves inside your veins become damaged, the valves may not close completely. This allows blood to flow in both directions. When your muscles relax, the valves inside the damaged vein(s) will not be able to hold the blood. This can cause pooling of blood or swelling in the veins. The veins bulge and appear as ropes under the skin. The blood begins to move more slowly through the veins, it may stick to the sides of the vessel walls and blood clots can form.

VARICOSE VEINS

These are bulging, swollen, purple, ropy veins, seen just under your skin, caused by damaged valves within the veins. They are more common in women than men and often run in families. They can also be caused by pregnancy, being severely overweight or by standing for long periods of time. The symptoms include bulging, swollen, purple, ropy, veins seen under the skin. Spider veins - small red or purple bursts on your knees, calves, or thighs, caused by swollen capillaries (small blood vessels). Aching, stinging, or swelling of the legs at the end of the day.

DEEP VEIN THROMBOSIS (DVT)

This is a blood clot occurring in a deep vein. When NBC News correspondent David Bloom died of a pulmonary embolism while covering the invasion of Baghdad, the term "deep vein thrombosis" (DVT) suddenly leaped into the headlines and public consciousness. DVT is caused by sitting in a constricted space for long periods. Most of us will never find ourselves living and sleeping for several days in an armored vehicle as David Bloom did, but every day, airline passengers who find themselves sitting in a cramped seat during a long flight experience the very sort of stresses that can prompt blood clotting in the legs. By some estimates, as many as 100,000 airline passengers may die from complications associated with DVT every year.

PULMONARY EMBOLISM

This is a blood clot (thrombus) that breaks loose from a leg or pelvic vein and travels to the pulmonary aretery of the lung. Most common following an operation, confinement to bed or deep vein thrombosis as mentioned above.

RISK FACTORS FOR CARDIOVASCULAR DISEASE

Determining heart-attack risk is a tricky thing because each of us has different susceptibility to cardiovascular disease. Some couch potatoes will live to 100 on fried chicken and milk shakes, while a few vegetarian marathon runners will suddenly drop dead of a heart attack at age 30. Your fitness level and diet do play a role in determining your chances of suffering a heart attack or stroke, but because cardiovascular disease is so common and silent, it is extremely important to recognize **all** the factors that put you at risk. These risk factors can be divided up into two categories: controllable (those you can do something about) and uncontrollable.

CONTROLLABLE RISK FACTORS

- **Cigarette smoking.** Smokers are more than twice as likely to have a heart attack than nonsmokers, and 2 to 4 times more likely to suffer sudden cardiac death. Tobacco smoke has about 4,000 toxic substances in it, any number of which can contribute to adverse effects on the blood vessels. Studies have shown that just one of these substances, nicotine, can cause plaque and tumors to grow much more quickly. Smoking also causes a decrease in the body's natural production of nitric oxide by as much as 50% for four hours. This is your body's natural defense against heart disease and stroke.

- **High cholesterol.** As cholesterol levels rise, so do your risks for cardiovascular disease. It is estimated that about 100 million Americans have high cholesterol levels. The major cause for the elevation in American cholesterol levels is the fast food, Western diet, which consists of an abundance of trans fatty acids and mountains of sugar.

- **High blood pressure.** High blood pressure causes the heart to work harder and, in time, weaken and enlarge. It also causes damage to the blood vessels because of the excessive pressure against the walls of the blood vessels.

- **Physical inactivity.** People who are sedentary are twice as likely to have a heart attack or stroke than people who are active. Regular, moderate to vigorous, exercise plays a role in protecting your cardiovascular health. Simply by taking a 30-minute vigorous walk everyday can add years to your life.

- **Obesity.** This disease (yes, it is a disease) is at epidemic proportions in the United States and may be the biggest reason why heart disease is our number one killer. People who are 35 pounds or more overweight tend to have increased blood pressure, higher cholesterol and fat levels, and higher sugar levels, which is the onset of diabetes. Add to this a more sedentary lifestyle and you can see how the cards are stacked against such a person.

- **Diabetes.** More than 25 to 30% of people with diabetes have vascular disease of the heart or limbs. This "silent epidemic" is characterized by high blood sugar levels which over time causes hardening of the arteries, which then leads to heart failure, kidney failure, blindness, or critical limb ischemia (amputation of a limb).

- **Stress.** Strong emotions stimulate the adrenal glands to release adrenaline into the blood steam. Adrenaline causes the heart to race, the blood vessels in the gut and skin to constrict, the blood vessels in the heart and brain to relax, and enhance the ability of the blood to clot. This explains how emotion can trigger chest pains while a person is having an anxiety attack. People under stress may also overeat, start smoking, or smoke more, which adds to your risk.

UNCONTROLLABLE RISK FACTORS

- **Age.** About 4 out of 5 people who die of heart disease are 65 or older. In fact, at this age, women are twice as likely to die from a heart attack than men. A woman lags behind a man by 10 years because her natural estrogen seems to protect her blood vessels. Once a woman reaches menopause, between the ages of 45 and 55, the incidence of coronary artery disease (CAD) spikes by as much as 400%. In fact, one out of two women will die of CAD and a 50 year old woman has a 10 times greater chance of dying from CAD than the combined risk from breast cancer and hip fracture.

- **Gender.** While it is generally believed that men have a greater risk of heart attack than women—and have heart attacks earlier in life—women are also at risk after they go through menopause. After menopause, generally a 10-year lag time behind men, women begin to catch up to me in terms of heart disease.

- **Race.** African-Americans, due to a tendency toward severe hypertension, diabetes and lack of vitamin D (because of the dark skin pigmentation) have twice the rate of heart disease than Caucasians.

- **Heredity.** The strongest risk factor for heart disease is a family history of heart attack or stroke at an early age (before the age of 55). Children of parents with heart disease are more likely to develop it themselves. If you have a family history of hardening of the arteries, you should be tested for homocysteine and lipoprotein (a), both of which are hereditary risk factors for heart disease.

- **Male Impotence.** If you are a man over 40 years old you might be feeling the effects of impotency. Researchers today know that upwards of 80% of impotence cases can be linked to purely physical problems. At this age our body begins to experience the results of poor diet and sedentary lifestyle. Science has discovered that high cholesterol, high blood pressure, diabetes, being over weight and smoking, not only are leading indicators for heart disease, but also are indicators for sexual dysfunction. In fact, so strong is the link between early impotence and atherosclerotic heart disease that some cardiologists have already begun considering impotence before age 60 as an early biomedical risk factor for heart disease. But you will soon find out in Chapter 6, that the same amino acid that can reverse the atherosclerotic heart and arteries, also has the ability to reverse sexual dysfunction in men and women. In fact, it is much more effective and safer than the Viagra type products.

CONCLUSION

If you have any one of these risk factors, it is likely your arteries are already showing signs of wear and tear; if you have two or three of these risk factors, your arteries are probably moderately impaired; if you have four or five of these risk factors, your arteries are probably severely impaired; and if you have more than five of theses risk factors, then you must know that you are living your life on a bubble and at any moment that bubble might burst.

The good news is, whatever the condition of your arteries, it is reversible and without taking powerful prescription drugs, through a natural protocol that I lay out for you in Chapter 6.

CHAPTER TWO
How Blood Pressure & Diabetes Affect The Heart

HYPERTENSION

---

52 million Americans suffer from elevated blood pressure levels, a silent condition called hypertension or high blood pressure. 45,000 Americans die every year from high blood pressure, costing the economy $50 billion per year. **Having high blood pressure raises your risk of having a heart attack by 3-fold, having heart failure by 4-fold and having a stroke by 7-fold.**

First, what is the cause of high blood pressure? In about 10% of cases there is a clearly established cause for high blood pressure, conditions such as renal artery stenosis, hyperthyroidism, or kidney problems. If these are treated, the blood pressure drops back to normal.

However, in about 90% of cases when the blood pressure is raised, no cause can be found. At which point, the medical profession, rather than using the term 'raised blood pressure of no known cause,' decided to rename the condition Essential Hypertension. You have got to admit, this sounds a great deal more scientific and 'disease like.' In fact, it sounds so impressive that Essential Hypertension has managed the transformation from a 'symptomless medical sign' to a real disease, one that needs to be treated.

Let us examine the logic in use here. One day, for no known reason, your body decides that the blood pressure needs to be raised. So your heart pumps harder, or your arteries decide to contract, or both. This has the desired effect of raising the blood pressure to a point where it can cause damage. It can lead to strokes, heart failure, kidney failure, etc.

Undeterred by the damage that this raised blood pressure is causing, the body continues day after day, month after month, year after year, to keep the pressure up. Eventually your heart cannot carry on any more, so it starts to pack in, you develop heart failure, and within about five years you are dead.

There is just one little thing missing from this model. A cause. Why does the pressure suddenly rise? One thing is for sure; the body does nothing without a cause, especially if the effect is to damage health. So we need to ask a deeper level question. What could cause the blood pressure to rise?

In order to understand this, you need only to the grasp the exceedingly simple concept that the pressure of liquid flowing through a pipe is a function of two variables. The first variable is the rate of flow of the liquid; the second is the diameter of the pipe. If you want to increase the pressure you must pump more fluid, or narrow the pipe.

Therefore, if your blood pressure goes up, for no known reason, one of two basic things is happening:

- The heart is pumping harder
- The diameter of the arteries has narrowed (causing the heart to pump harder to keep the blood flow the same)

Things that make your heart pump harder would include: anxiety, inflammation, exercise, and stimulants, e.g. coffee. Things that narrow your arteries would be atherosclerotic plaque (the underlying cause of coronary artery disease) would narrow an artery. Therefore, a probable cause of high blood pressure is the presence of coronary artery disease.

Thus, high blood pressure is not a cause of coronary heart disease. Instead coronary heart disease is a cause of high blood pressure. So yet again, as with raised cholesterol levels and coronary heart disease, we see another rather grisly example of the medical profession grasping the wrong end of the stick and desperately trying to cure coronary heart disease by sweeping a symptom of that disease (high blood pressure) under the carpet. No big surprise, it does not actually work.

Does this all seem incredibly basic? It should, because it is. So, while blood pressure lowering may have some effect on preventing strokes, heart failure and other pressure related problems, it has no effect on reducing death from heart attacks. After all, how could it?

Your blood pressure is the result of a complex system that includes not only your heart and blood vessels, but also hormones and protein messengers. As your heart pumps, it sends blood through your arteries. Healthy arteries expand under the pressure then contract when the pressure wave passes; however, inelastic arteries (arterioscleosis) cannot expand, and high pressure is created when blood pumps.

Blood pressure refers to the force of blood pushing against the chambers of the heart and walls of the arteries as it is pumped and circulated throughout the body. When blood pressure is too high, the excessive force of blood against the arteries causes their cellular walls to become weak and porous, which is an open invitation to toxic substances such as cholesterol to take up residence on their smooth muscle lining. This is why high blood pressure is a major contributor to coronary artery disease, specifically stroke, heart attack, and congestive heart failure.

High blood pressure increases your risks of dying from a heart attack by three-fold, heart failure by four-fold, and stroke by seven-fold.

Receptors in your kidneys keep track of the pressure and send hormone signals telling your heart to speed up or slow down as needed. Readings that are consistently above 150/90 are a risk factor for the heart.

Blood pressure measurement involves two key numbers: systolic—the pressure in your arteries when your heart is pumping, and diastolic—the pressure when your heart is at rest between beats. A healthy reading is within the range of 120-130 over 80-85. A borderline reading is around 140/90. High blood pressure (hypertension) is anything over 150/85.

It is estimated that 52 million of us have high blood pressure, making it the #1 condition that cardiologists and internists treat today. Of this number, some three-quarters are on prescription medication to control their hypertension. These drugs can be lifesavers, but they can also cause a host of unpleasant side effects—impotence, loss of sexual desire, fatigue, drowsiness, dry cough, lightheadedness, and even depression. **Remember: You can increase your chances of living a longer, healthier life if you can decrease your reliance on drugs.**

ACCURACY IS KEY WHEN MEASURING BLOOD PRESSURE

Blood pressure readings are like the Dow Jones average; they go up and down, even in a five-minute interval. Remember, your heart is a pulsating, dynamic organ, so your blood pressure can vary sometimes as much as 20 to 30 mm in successive readings. The following are some tips to accurately measure one's blood pressure.

- First of all, the worst place to take a blood pressure reading is in a doctor's office. Most people enter a doctor's office with considerable anxiety (called hyperarousal) about their blood pressure, and that drives the numbers up. Try to relax by taking a couple of deep breaths.

- Also be aware that simple daily things like being rushed, caught in traffic, coming in from cold temperatures, having emotional stress, or having a cup of coffee or tea just prior to the test can drive the numbers up.

- Make sure that your blood pressure is taken in a proper fashion. In one study, 73% of health professionals failed to use proper arm and cuff positions. The standards established by the *American Heart Association* call for patients undergoing blood pressure readings to be seated with their back supported, and their bare arm resting on a table so the cuff is placed at the upper portion of the arm considered to be at "heart level." An investigation by the *Annals of Internal Medicine* found that blood pressure readings were 9-14 mm higher when the arm was positioned parallel to the torso. Finally, the patient's feet should be on the floor and no clothing should be on the arm, as this may give an erroneous reading.

- Taking one's blood pressure at home is the best way to obtain accurate numbers. First, a person is more relaxed, and second, the best way to accurately know your blood pressure is to take several readings during a 24-hour period and then average them out.

CONTROLLABLE RISK FACTORS FOR HIGH BLOOD PRESSURE

- **Poor diet.** A diet high in animal protein and animal fats contributes to clogged or hardened arteries, forcing your heart to pump harder to push blood through.

- **Too much salt.** Salt is a problem for people who are salt-sensitive—most notably African and Native Americans and thus they should restrict the amount of their daily intake of salt.

Mainstream medicine tells us that **all** patients with hypertension should avoid salt in their diets. But recently this idea has been questioned, and often dismissed by many doctors.

For instance, according to the late Robert C. Atkins, M.D., author of "Dr. Atkins' Diet Revolution," the problem for those with high blood pressure is not sodium; it is a lack of balance between sodium and potassium levels.

Dr. Atkins cites the results of 30 separate studies that show how increasing potassium intake (without decreasing the sodium) is an effective way to lower blood pressure. One of those studies demonstrated that with just one daily serving of a potassium-rich food the risk of death by stroke may be cut by as much as half.

The good news: It is easy to increase the potassium in your diet. High potassium fruits include apricots, bananas, cantaloupe, honeydew melon and citrus fruits. Vegetables with good amounts of potassium are asparagus, potatoes, green beans, avocados, lima beans, winter squash, and cauliflower. Other foods high in potassium: grain products, red meat, poultry, seafood and dry beans, such as peas and lentils.

Salt, without a balance of potassium, can increase the volume of your blood, causing blood vessels to expand and the pressure to rise. This is a big burden on your heart. High levels of salt are hidden in processed foods: canned vegetables, powdered soups, dips, diet soft drinks and preserved meats such as bacon and sausage. A single dill pickle can contain as much as 1000 mg of salt. Keep your daily intake within the range of 2000 to 3000 mg. Try using trace-mineral-rich sea salt rather than over processed plain table salt.

- **Excess weight and sedentary lifestyle.** In one study, three out of four patients with high blood pressure achieved normal blood pressure with no drug therapy, after losing a specific amount of weight. Losing even 10% of your body weight can have a significant effect on lowering your blood pressure. A study by the *National Institute of Health* revealed that just by walking one to two miles a day could save the lives of more than 150,000 people each year.

- **Unresolved anger, high-stress lifestyle, and "workaholism"** can contribute to high blood pressure.

- **Smoking.** Hypertensive smokers are three times more likely than nonsmokers to suffer strokes, and twice as likely to suffer a heart attack. Smoking constricts your blood vessels, which in turn raises your blood pressure.

- **Syndrome X, insulin resistance (hyperinsulinemia).** This is a complex of factors resulting from eating too many refined sugars and starches (carbohydrates), which leads to excess insulin production. Eventually, your insulin receptors shut down, preventing glucose—your body's chief energy source—from entering your cells. What happens? You are hungry all the time for carbohydrates, but at the same time, you have little energy—you are mentally and physically exhausted, even when you are relatively inactive. Over time, you will be at a high risk for high blood pressure, thickened arteries and even Type II, non-insulin-dependent diabetes. Stay away from diets that promote low fat and high carbohydrates, it would be like throwing gasoline on a fire!

- **Heavy drinking.** Consuming more than one or two alcoholic beverages per day increases blood pressure an average of 10 mm/Hg. Try only one drink per day for women and two drinks per day for men.

- **Over reliance on anti-inflammatory medications.** Studies show that ibuprofen (i.e. Motrin, Advil) and Naproxen (i.e. Aleve) raise blood pressure by an average of 3.5 mm/Hg to 10 mm/Hg. Antihistamines and other over-the-counter cold remedies can contribute to high blood pressure. Fortunately, aspirin appears to have little or no effect on blood pressure or salt retention.

- **White-coat syndrome.** It is a proven fact that many folks' blood pressure shoots up in the doctor's office. When the doctor or nurse walks in and straps that cuff around your arm, your heart begins to beat faster, and before you know it, your blood pressure is skyrocketing.

THE MEDICAL ECONOMICS OF HYPERTENSION

With high blood pressure existing in one out of every three American adults, it is clear that pharmacological management of hypertension pulls in big bucks. According to a recent article in the *Journal of the American Medical Association,* "Treatment of hypertension has become the leading reason for visits to physicians as well as drug prescriptions."

Close to $9 billion dollars a year is being spent to treat hypertension. This figure includes neither the dollars spent on medications prescribed to mask the side effects of antihypertensive drugs nor the increased price of treating heart attacks and strokes associated with these antihypertensive drugs, which cost the nation another $8 billion dollars a year.

Despite substantial evidence that lifestyle changes alone can in many cases reduce blood pressure, antihypertensive drugs are still the most common form of conventional treatment. Please read the next section for natural ways to combat high blood pressure and further in Chapter 5 in this book for the types of drugs used and their negative side effects.

NATURAL WAYS TO LOWER BLOOD PRESSURE

Dietary Modifications

- The Mediterranean diet is so named because it is similar to the diet of people living near the Mediterranean Sea. Researchers found that people living in seven countries adjacent to the Mediterranean Sea had one-third to one-quarter the death rate from heart disease than those living in the northern regions of Europe. The Mediterranean diet consists of more whole grains, more root and green vegetables, more fruit, more fish, less red meat (replaced with chicken), and butter is replaced with canola oil and olive oil for salads and food preparation.

- Cardia Salt contains 50 percent less sodium per serving. The sodium is replaced by potassium, magnesium and lysine, all of which will help maintain a normal heartbeat and reduce blood pressure. If you must have salt, try not to exceed more than 2,000-3,000 mg per day.

- High potassium/magnesium snacks, such as bananas, figs, pumpkin seeds, kiwi, mango, blueberries, grapes (fresh or dried, without sulfites)

- Carrot juice—one 6-oz glass a day

- Green tea—two cups a day, not after 2 p.m. because it contains caffeine

Targeted Nutritional Supplements

- Arginine—5-6 grams per day (read in Chapter 6 how arginine helps to lower blood pressure)

- Calcium/magnesium in 2.5:1 ratio—1200/500 mg per day

- Coenzyme Q10—150-300 mg/day

- Hawthorne berry—up to 1500 mg/day

- Garlic—1 small clove or one capsule a day

- Grape seed extract—300 mg/day

- Tumeric (curcumin)—500 mg/day

Lifestyle Modifications

- Daily exercise, such as walking

- Weight loss—increase in lean body mass (BMI)

- Quit smoking

- Limit alcohol intake—two drinks per day for men and one drink per day for women

Emotional Healing, Anger and Stress Control

Meditation	Yoga
Bioenergetics	Tai Chi
Prayer	Biofeedback
Music	Touch therapy
Deep breathing	Having a pet
Dance	

DIABETES MELLITUS

According to the latest figures from the *Centers for Disease Control and Prevention (CDC)*, nearly **21 million Americans have diabetes mellitus**, which is commonly referred to as diabetes. That is 7% of the American population. About 6 million of those people have no idea they have diabetes and millions more are at risk of developing it. If you have diabetes, your body has problems converting the food you eat into energy.

The danger of this lies in the fact that if untreated, diabetes can damage the eyes, kidneys, nerves, heart and blood vessels. Therefore, whenever present, it is essential to diagnose, monitor and treat diabetes correctly.

Diabetes mellitus should not be confused with diabetes insipidus (DI). Diabetes insipidus and diabetes mellitus are unrelated, although they can have similar signs and symptoms, like excessive thirst and excessive urination.

INSULIN AND BLOOD SUGAR

Normally, the food we eat is broken down into glucose, which is a form of sugar. The glucose passes into the bloodstream where it is used by cells for growth and energy. For cells to use glucose, however, insulin must be present. Insulin is a hormone produced by the pancreas, a large gland behind the stomach. If the insulin is not present, or if the cells do not respond to it, the glucose stays in the bloodstream, causing a rise in the blood sugar or blood glucose level. When blood sugar levels are too high it is called hyperglycemia; when blood sugar levels fall too low it is called hypoglycemia. The *National Institute of Diabetes and Digestive and Kidney Diseases (NIDDK)* says conditions that can lead to hypoglycemia in people with diabetes include taking too much medication, missing or delaying a meal, eating too little food for the amount of insulin taken, exercising too strenuously, drinking too much alcohol, or any combination of these factors.

TYPES OF DIABETES

The American Diabetes Association (ADA) and *NIDDK* say there are different types of diabetes and insulin-resistance:

Type 1 diabetes, also called insulin-dependent or immune-mediated diabetes, occurs when your body cannot produce insulin. This is the kind of diabetes that often appears before the age of 18, although it can also strike at any age. Type 1 diabetes is considered an autoimmune disease. An autoimmune disease results when the body's system for fighting infection, the immune system, turns against a part of the body. In Type 1 diabetes, according to *NIDDK,* the immune system attacks the insulin-producing cells in the pancreas and destroys them. The pancreas then produces little or no insulin. An individual with Type 1 diabetes requires daily doses of insulin. The insulin can be delivered by injection, through a pump system, which feeds the insulin into the body through a needle or catheter inserted just under the skin or via an inhaler. Healthy meal planning and regular exercise are also a part of the treatment for Type 1 diabetes.

Type 2 diabetes, also called non-insulin-dependent diabetes and adult on-set diabetes, is much more common than Type 1 diabetes, affecting some 95% of people with diabetes and amazingly half are unaware that they even have this disease. In this type, your body *can* produce insulin, but it either does not produce enough or it is not using it properly. For a while their bodies attempt to make more insulin to make up for the resistance. But after a while, their production cannot keep up with the increased insulin resistance and blood sugar rises. The initial treatment is dieting to help maintain or lose weight, but often this will not be enough and will lead to medication followed by insulin injections.

Type 2 diabetes has been linked with obesity and the number of people in the U.S. with both obesity and Type 2 diabetes is growing.

In fact, there is alarming news from the *Center for Disease Control and Prevention (CDC)*, whose numbers are showing that Type 2 diabetes, which affected just adults (age 45 an older), is now growing among younger adults and teenagers like never before and are now calling it a "silent epidemic!" I wonder if our children's fast food diets of empty carbohydrates, excess sodium and sugar, and trans fatty acids might have anything to do with this increase. Would you like to "super size" that order?

PRE-DIABETES

The U.S. Department of Health and Human Services (HHS) says there is also a condition called "pre-diabetes" which affects an additional 41 million Americans. The term "pre-diabetes" is being used to describe an increasingly common condition in which blood glucose levels are higher than normal but not yet diabetic. This is also known as impaired glucose tolerance or impaired fasting glucose. Someone with impaired glucose tolerance may also be described as "insulin resistant," that is, their body produces insulin but is not utilizing it correctly, causing blood sugar levels to rise.

Insulin resistance is also a factor in metabolic syndrome or syndrome X. Other risk factors for metabolic syndrome include a body mass index of over 25, high triglyceride levels, family history of diabetes, polycystic ovary syndrome, sedentary lifestyle, age and ethnicity. *The American College of Endocrinology (ACE)* and the *American Association of Clinical Endocrinologists (AACE)* say metabolic syndrome is an epidemic condition that dramatically increases risk for Type 2 diabetes, heart disease and stroke.

They estimate that it affects one in three Americans. *HHS* says most people with pre-diabetes will likely develop diabetes within a decade unless they make changes in their diet and level of physical activity, which can help them reduce their risks. Even before they develop diabetes, their health is still at risk, since they are much more likely to develop high blood pressure, abnormal blood lipids and coronary heart disease. Studies have linked obesity to impaired glucose tolerance, as well as to pre-diabetes.

SYMPTOMS OF DIABETES

Symptoms of diabetes can vary, but the *American Academy of Family Physicians* says typical symptoms include:

- Frequent urination

- Excessive thirst
- Blurry vision
- Tingling or numbness in the hands and feet
- Unexplained weight loss despite eating more than usual
- Extreme tiredness or irritability

HEART DISEASE AND STROKE

The *American Heart Association (AHA)* says diabetes is also a major risk factor for stroke, coronary heart disease and heart attack. According to *AHA,* two-thirds of people with diabetes mellitus die of some form of heart or blood vessel disease, and adults with diabetes are two to four times more likely to have heart disease or suffer a stroke than adults without diabetes. Patients who have suffered from diabetes since childhood, especially if it has been poorly controlled, are at significant risk of developing one of these life-threatening problems as early as their 20's or 30's. *AHA* says insulin resistance, a condition where the body cannot use the insulin it produces effectively and a key component of Type 2 diabetes, is associated with blood lipid imbalances, such as an increased ratio of small low-density lipoprotein (LDL or so-called bad cholesterol), low levels of high-density lipoprotein (HDL or so-called good cholesterol), and increased levels of triglycerides, all of which are linked to higher risk of heart disease.

AHA adds that people with diabetes may avoid or delay heart and blood vessel disease by controlling both their diabetes as well as the risk factors associated with heart disease. However, studies show many people with diabetes are unaware of their increased risk of heart disease and the importance of taking steps to reduce their risk by careful monitoring of blood sugar levels combined with weight loss, blood pressure and cholesterol control, and not smoking.

People who have diabetes tend to get a particularly bad form of atherosclerosis because it tends to affect the smaller, as well as larger, vessels. In fact new studies show that anyone over 50, who is also a diabetic, has an 80% chance of developing peripheral arterial disease

(PAD). Like the blood vessels of the heart (coronary arteries), your peripheral arteries (blood vessels outside your heart) also may develop atherosclerosis, the build-up of fat and cholesterol deposits, called plaque, on the inside walls. Over time, the build-up narrows the artery. Eventually the narrowed artery causes less blood to flow and a condition called "ischemia" can occur. Ischemia is inadequate blood flow to the body's tissue. A blockage in the legs can lead to leg pain or cramps with activity (a condition called claudication), changes in skin color, sores or ulcers and feeling tired in the legs. However, this can eventually lead to a total loss of circulation, which can then lead to gangrene and amputation.

FACING THE FUTURE

Anyone who has diabetes should have two basic goals: to reduce their reliance on prescribed medications and to reduce their risk of diabetic complications such as blindness, kidney failure, heart attack, and amputation of legs.

For someone with Type 1 or insulin-dependent diabetes, whose pancreas produces too little insulin, it is likely that insulin replacement will be necessary for the rest of his or her life. For people with this type diabetes, the object is not so much to get off insulin, but to prevent the long-term complications of diabetes mellitus. The amount of insulin needed can be reduced through appropriate diet, exercise and nutritional supplements, and the likelihood of complications will also be significantly decreased on this regime.

For someone with Type 2 or non-insulin-dependent diabetes, the object is to prevent future insulin dependency and currently reduce or even stop oral prescription drugs through appropriate diet, exercise and nutritional supplements. The major studies on these oral drugs, including DiaBeta, Glucotrol and Glucophage have shown that they actually increase the death rate from heart attacks. In fact, the warnings on these drugs in the *Physicians Desk Reference* state exactly that. The listed side effects for these drugs include increased risk of fatal heart attack, nausea, diarrhea, flatulence, bloating, photosensitivity, hives, skin eruptions and rash, itching, drowsiness, headache, metallic taste and loss of appetite.

NATURAL WAYS TO CONTROL BLOOD SUGAR

Dietary Modifications

- **Restricting all grains and sugars from the diet** is the most basic change a diabetic can do.

- **Replace fat calories with slow-burning carbohydrates.** Since the 1930s, numerous studies have shown that patients could stop taking insulin if they were given high-carbohydrate diets. And in 1976, Dr. James Anderson, from the *University of Kentucky*, demonstrated that the high-complex carbohydrate, high fiber diet could eliminate the need for insulin and oral diabetic drugs in close to 70 percent of diabetic patients. Most of a diabetics diet should consist of vegetables and legumes.

- **Eat adequate amounts of lean protein at every meal.**

- **Avoid processed foods**. Such as refined baked goods containing simple carbohydrates, which increase blood sugar, and starchy carbohydrates like, breads, potatoes, corn and white rice.

- **Avoid saturated fats,** which block the effect of insulin. Replace with healthy fats like, raw nuts and seeds, flax, olive and canola oil.

- **Eat fruits sparingly.** Although they are very good for you, they are also high in fruit sugars.

- **Add cinnamon to your diet**. Adding a spoonful of cinnamon per day to your diet can work wonders in regulating your blood sugar. What makes cinnamon effective in managing and preventing diabetes is a flavonoid called methylhydroxychalcone polymer (MHCP) that closely mimics insulin activity. In several studies, Dr. Richard Anderson and a team of researchers at *Iowa State University* found that a combination of MHCP and insulin worked synergistically in regulating glucose metabolism, and further, that MHCP can work alone without the presence of insulin as well.

Lifestyle Modifications

- **Daily exercise**, such as walking. Exercise works by increasing the sensitivity of insulin receptors so the insulin that is present works more effectively and your body does not need to produce as much. Research shows low intensity aerobic activity, like walking works fine. And engaging in this activity after eating is best, since glucose levels rise after meals.

- **Weight loss**. About 80% of people with diabetes are also significantly overweight. There is also a strong relationship between Type 2 diabetes and depression, but whether the depression is brought on by the diabetes or obesity or both remains unclear.

- **Quit smoking**

- **Limit alcohol intake**—two drinks per day for men and one drink per day for women.

Targeted Nutritional Supplements

The biggest oversight of the current medical approach to diabetes is its failure to recognize that diabetes is a nutritional wasting disease. An elevated blood sugar level acts as an osmotic diuretic, which explains why diabetics experience increased urination. More important, diabetes causes massive losses of nutrients, like vitamins B-1, B-6, and B12, and the minerals magnesium, zinc and chromium to name a few.

This loss of nutrients obviously contributes to, and could be the primary reason for, the deterioration of the eyes, kidneys, peripheral nerves and blood vessels, which often occurs with diabetes. You cannot get the proper level of nutrients from diet alone.

- **Arginine** 5000 mg. Many published clinical studies support how arginine can prevent diabetes, reverses damage caused by diabetes, reduces insulin resistance and improves blood sugar disposal in diabetes mellitus Type 2 patients. More about arginine and diabetes in Chapter 6.

- **Magnesium** 750 mg. 90% of diabetics have magnesium deficiency. Insulin and oral drugs have been shown to deplete magnesium from a diabetics' body.

- **Chromium Picolonate** 400 mcg. Chromium enhances your body's sensitivity to insulin and reduces complications by lowering blood glucose levels.

- **Gymnema Sylvestre** 500 mg. This extract of the leaves of a central and south India plant, has been shown to lower blood sugar and may help repair the pancreas.

- **Vanadyl Sulfate** 100 mg. This is a form of the trace mineral vanadium that has proven extremely effective in reducing the need for insulin in diabetics. In large doses, vanadyl sulfate works remarkably like oral insulin; in fact, better. In experimental animals, it has completely eliminated diabetes permanently, even after the vanadyl sulfate was stopped.

- **Biotin** 2 mg. Biotin is part of the complex of B vitamins and has been shown to help metabolize fats, proteins and carbohydrates. According to the *Linus Pauling Institute (LPI)*, biotin research on rats indicates that this vitamin may stimulate insulin secretion in the pancreas.

- **Vitamin B Complex.** One of the first nutrition zingers I ever read was Dr. Carlton Fredericks comment (in *Food Facts and Fallacies*) to the effect that diabetics could be weaned off of insulin with extremely high doses of B-complex vitamins. I am a conservative person and I have my sincere doubts if a Type 1 diabetic could ever be free of the need to take insulin. On the other hand, I have personally seen diabetics require significantly less insulin when they take a 100 mg balanced B-complex tablet every two to three hours. The potential benefits are so great that I think diabetics should demand a suitably cautious therapeutic trial of megavitamin therapy with insulin dosage adjustments made and supervised by their physician.

- **Vitamin C** 2500 mg. Physicians investigated the effects of 2000 mg/day of vitamin C on a group of 56 non-insulin-dependent diabetics. The vitamin C improved control of blood sugar and fasting blood-sugar levels. It also lowered cholesterol and triglyceride levels, and reduced capillary fragility. In fact, reviews of medical literature as far back as 1940 show that blood sugar could be predictably reduced with intravenous ascorbate vitamin C.

- **Vitamin E** 1200 IU. In a crossover study on 36 patients who had Type 1 diabetes for less than 10 years, the dose evaluated was 1800 I.U. per day. Before taking vitamin E, retinal blood flows in these subjects was significantly lower than in the non-diabetic population. Both retinal blood flow and creatine clearance were significantly normalized when subjects received vitamin E. ***The patients with the worst reading improved the most.*** The vitamin had no effect on blood glucose levels, and therefore will not interfere with insulin therapy.

Making these changes in your lifestyle will help to optimize your insulin levels. As some people may know, blood sugar is only the symptom in most diabetics; the real challenge is to control your insulin levels. Once the insulin levels are stabilized, it is common for the blood sugar to come back to normal levels. Along with controlling your diabetes, these basic lifestyle changes will also lead to several inevitable side effects like increasing your energy and normalizing your weight, so getting started today will likely lead to an increased quality of life on many different levels.

CHAPTER THREE
Causes of Heart Disease

Once upon a time, doctors and scientists blamed cholesterol as the cause for heart disease. Today people are exercising like crazy, changing their diets, gulping handfuls of supplements, and 30% of Americans over 55 are taking expensive statin drugs to lower their cholesterol. Yet none of this is making a dent in heart attack statistics and not one study has been able to show that these drugs do anything to lengthen a person's lifespan.

Some doctors and scientists are finally having second thoughts about cholesterol's role in heart disease. They have discovered that cholesterol is only one piece of the cardiac-risk pie, and may be a very small piece at that.

We will begin by looking at cholesterol's role in causing heart disease and then continue looking at the other pieces of the cardiac-risk pie. Having the knowledge of the many contributing factors for heart disease is a beginning to reversing its deadly grip or preventing it from ever happening to yourself or someone you love.

CHOLESTEROL

Not long ago, scientists believed high cholesterol was at the root of heart disease, and that consumption of a high-fat, high cholesterol diet led to the plaque buildup on artery walls, setting the stage for a heart attack. The truth is that cholesterol is **NOT** the deadly threat you think it is!

It is, in fact, the most important molecule in your body. Cholesterol gives structure to every cell in the body much like the two by fours in a house. Aside from the fact that it is necessary for everything from the production of sex hormones to bile synthesis...it does not clog your arteries unless it has something to attach to; a tear, a rough surface, a ridge, a sharp turn.

Hypercholesterolemia is the health issue of the 21st century. **It is actually an invented disease**, a "problem" that emerged when health professionals learned how to measure cholesterol levels in the blood. High cholesterol exhibits no outward signs--unlike other conditions of the blood, such as diabetes or anemia, diseases that manifest telltale symptoms like thirst or weakness--hypercholesterolemia requires the services of a physician to detect its presence. Many people who feel perfectly healthy suffer from high cholesterol--in fact, feeling good is actually a symptom of high cholesterol!

Doctors who treat this new disease must first convince their patients that they are sick and need to take one or more expensive drugs for the rest of their lives, drugs that require regular checkups and blood tests. But such doctors do not work in a vacuum--their efforts to convert healthy people into patients are bolstered by the full weight of the U.S. government, the media and the medical establishment, agencies that have worked in concert to disseminate the cholesterol dogma and convince the population that high cholesterol is the forerunner of heart disease and possibly other diseases as well.

Who suffers from hypercholesterolemia? Peruse the medical literature of 25 or 30 years ago and you'll get the following answer: any middle-aged man whose cholesterol is over 240 with other risk factors, such as smoking or overweight.

After the Cholesterol Consensus Conference in 1984, the parameters changed; **anyone** with cholesterol over 200 could receive the dreaded diagnosis and a prescription for pills. Recently that number has been moved down to 180. If you have had a heart attack, you get to take cholesterol-lowering medicines even if your cholesterol is already very low--after all, you have committed the sin of having a heart attack so your cholesterol must therefore be too high. The penance is a lifetime of cholesterol-lowering medications along with a boring low-fat diet. But why wait until you have a heart attack? Current edicts stipulate cholesterol testing and treatment for young adults and even children.

New research at leading medical centers, including Harvard, are now saying that cholesterol is guilty by association because more than 60% of heart attack victims actually have normal cholesterol levels and the majority of people with high cholesterol never suffer heart attacks. In fact, 50% of heart attack victims have none of the standard risk factors listed by the *American Heart Association.*

The cholesterol theory was brought into question when researchers discovered that one particular type of cholesterol, high-density lipoprotein (HDL) cholesterol, actually has a protective effect on the heart; and that lipoprotein(a) (Lp(a)), a low-density lipoprotein (LDL), is a sticky protein, which adheres to artery walls, is actually the culprit.

We now know that cholesterol contributes to heart disease **only** when it is oxidized, or subjected to free radical damage. Cholesterol damaged by free radicals is taken up by white blood cells called macrophages and deposited in fatty streaks on the artery walls. This fosters plaque buildup in the arteries and is key in the development of heart disease. If one can stop the oxidation process, then one can eliminate cholesterol from the picture.

Nowhere is the failing of our medical system more evident than in the wholesale acceptance of cholesterol reduction as a way to prevent disease. Have all these doctors forgotten what they learned in Biochemistry 101 about the many roles of cholesterol in the human biochemistry?

Every cell membrane in our body contains cholesterol because cholesterol is what makes our cells waterproof--without cholesterol we could not have a different biochemistry on the inside and the outside of the cell. When cholesterol levels are not adequate, the cell membrane becomes leaky or porous, a situation the body interprets as an emergency, releasing a flood of corticoid hormones that work by sequestering cholesterol from one part of the body and transporting it to areas where it is lacking. Cholesterol is the body's repair substance: scar tissue contains high levels of cholesterol, including scar tissue in the arteries.

Cholesterol is the precursor to vitamin D, necessary for numerous biochemical processes including mineral metabolism. The bile salts, required for the digestion of fat, are made of cholesterol. Those who suffer from low cholesterol often have trouble digesting fats. Cholesterol also functions as a powerful antioxidant, thus protecting us against cancer and aging.

Cholesterol is vital to proper neurological function. It plays a key role in the formation of memory and the uptake of hormones in the brain, including serotonin, the body's feel-good chemical. When cholesterol levels drop too low, the serotonin receptors cannot work. Cholesterol is the main organic molecule in the brain, constituting over half the dry weight of the cerebral cortex.

Finally, cholesterol is the precursor to all the hormones produced in the adrenal cortex including glucocorticoids, which regulate blood sugar levels, and mineralocorticoids, which regulate mineral balance. Corticoids are the cholesterol-based adrenal hormones that the body uses in response to stress of various types; it promotes healing and balances the tendency to inflammation. The adrenal cortex also produces sex hormones out of cholesterol, including testosterone, estrogen and progesterone. Thus, low cholesterol, whether due to an innate error of metabolism or induced by cholesterol-lowering diets and drugs, can be expected to disrupt the production of adrenal hormones and lead to: blood sugar problems, edema, allergies, asthma, mineral deficiencies, reduced libido, chronic inflammation, infertility, difficulty in healing, and various reproductive problems.

In its natural state cholesterol is waxy and doesn't mix with your blood. It must combine with other proteins to form HDL (beneficial) and LDL (harmful). One of HDL's functions is to scavenge LDL and transport it to the liver for breakdown. Your body can do this, but the process requires nutrients that are often missing from modern diets.

High cholesterol levels (consistently above 225 total) are considered a risk for heart disease. You need to reduce LDL and raise HDL levels so that your ratio of LDL to HDL is lower than 5:1. Your LDL is to be no more than 180 mg/dl (ideally 160) and ideally, your HDL should be 60 mg/dl or greater. At a minimum, men should be at 35 mg/dl and women at 45 mg/dl or more. Research shows that the risk for coronary heart disease is 2.5 times greater when HDL cholesterol falls below 35 mg/dl.

Here is an interesting fact—the cholesterol in your diet has very little effect on the cholesterol in your blood. You could completely eliminate all cholesterol from your diet and your liver would just produce more. On the other hand, eating more cholesterol would cause your liver to reduce production to maintain consistent levels.

Natural remedies to lower LDL cholesterol while raising HDL cholesterol include: the Mediterranean diet, exercise (regular physical exercise raises "good" HDL), arginine, niacin, polycosanol, tocotrienols, omega-3 and omega-6 fatty acids, flax and fiber, probiotics, coenzyme Q10, magnesium, vitamin E, lecithin, garlic and DHEA; more about these natural therapies in Chapter 6.

I know many of you are asking yourselves, but what about the drug I am taking to lower my cholesterol? We will discuss these drugs in depth in Chapter 5 of this book, but for now you might find it interesting to learn that in 1968, Dr. Kilmer McCully, Dean of Medicine at the *University of New York*, published a report saying that heart disease was caused by homocysteine, that cholesterol was not the crucial marker for heart disease that everyone thought it was, and that cholesterol drugs were not necessary. Well in 1968 the cholesterol drug industry was a 7 billion dollar a year industry, and let us not forget about the other 20 billion dollars spent on drugs to counteract the negative side effects of the cholesterol drugs. Just three weeks after his report was published he lost his tenure to teach, and shortly after that he lost his license to practice medicine. After all, whom did he think he was making such claims! It was not until 30 years later, in 1998, that he was finally vindicated. He was nominated for two *Nobel* prizes for his research, he was re-instated as Dean of Medicine at the *University of New York*, he was given his medical license back, and he was given the task of teaching doctors that cholesterol is not the cause of heart disease; more on Dr. McCully's homocysteine theory and use of cholesterol drugs later in this book.

Now let us begin to look at the other pieces of the cardiac-risk pie, which are Homocysteine, C-Reactive Protein (CRP), Lipoprotein A (LP(a)), and Fibrinogen.

HOMOCYSTEINE

Kilmer McCully, M.D., discovered the homocysteine/heart disease link in 1968. Dr. McCully had learned about homocystinuria, a newly discovered disease, at a medical conference. He found that mentally retarded youngsters had often been found to have the chemical homocysteine in their urine. These children died from a condition indistinguishable from hardening of the arteries in the elderly.

Researchers found that homocyseine was also in the blood of adults. The question in Dr. McCully's mind was, does the level of the chemical homocysteine in the blood correlate with hardening of the arteries? Is it possible that the fat and cholesterol deposits seen in arteriosclerotic arterial plaques are only secondary accretions after homocysteine has already done the damage? The answer he soon discovered was yes, and in 1968 he announced the homocysteine theory of heart disease. In essence, Dr. McCully announced to the world at that time that the cholesterol theory was a hoax and a delusion, that cholesterol does not cause arteriosclerosis, and that the elevation of blood cholesterol is a symptom—not a cause of heart disease.

Today there is a growing consensus that homocysteine may be a major contributor to degenerative diseases such as artheroscerosis. Over the years, studies have shown that an elevated blood level of homocysteine is a highly predictable risk factor for heart disease. In fact, a recent *Harvard* study of 271 patients has confirmed that **men with high homocysteine levels are 300% more likely to have a heart attack** than the rest of the population.

Elevated homocysteine levels have also been named as the prime suspect in causing a large list of health related issues, including many age-related heart and brain problems, cognitive difficulties, deep vein thrombosis, moodiness, intermittent claudication (leg pain), low birth weight, bone loss, poor circulation, and a multiple of cardiovascular difficulties.

Homocysteine often causes the initial lesions on arterial walls that enable (LDL) cholesterol and fibrinogen to accumulate and eventually to obstruct blood flow. Homocysteine also contributes to the oxidation of LDL cholesterol and the accumulation of arterial plaque and subsequent vascular blockage. Homocysteine damages cells directly by promoting oxidative stress. It will turn the walls of your healthy blood vessels into rusty pipes. Homocysteine also can cause abnormal arterial blood clots (thrombosis) that can completely block an artery.

Homocysteine alone has been demonstrated to promote artheroscleosis and thrombosis, even if cholesterol and triglyceride levels are not significantly elevated.

Recent research informs us that women whose blood pressure and homocysteine levels are both elevated have 25 times the incidence of vascular events, including stroke or heart attack.

New studies from *Harvard* and published in the *New England Journal of Medicine* show there can be little doubt: If you want to dramatically slash your risk of heart disease, you must lower your high levels of homocysteine.

Your body forms homocysteine when you eat food containing an amino acid called methionine, which is present in all animal and vegetable protein. As part of the digestive process, methionine is broken down into homocysteine. As long as certain helper nutrients are present, homocysteine subsequently converts back into one of two harmless amino acids. However, lack of these helper nutrients leaves us with poor methylation (detoxification of harmful compounds), which causes an excess of homocysteine to spill out of our cells and into our bloodstream where it damages the arteries, setting the stage for the buildup of plaque in our arteries.

These helper nutrients are vitamins B6, B12 and most importantly folic acid (folate). Unfortunately, the typical American diet of processed foods is low in these helper nutrients and high in methionine. The problem with processed foods is not only the omission of B vitamins, but the fact that processed foods actually deplete the body of B vitamins, which is a double negative.

Homocysteine levels can be accurately determined in a blood test. If your homocysteine levels are low (6-8 micromoles per liter), you are at low risk of developing heart disease, but epidemiological evidence suggests that optimal levels are less than 8 micromoles per liter and levels above 20 micromoles per liter quadruple your risk of heart attack.

The following people especially need to test their homocysteine levels: If you have had a heart attack or other cardiovascular event; if you have a family history of early heart disease; if you have hypothyroidism; if you have lupus or kidney disease; and if you take drugs that tend to elevate homocysteine levels—niacin (for cholesterol lowering), theophylline (for asthma), methotrexate (for cancer or arthritis), or L-dopa (for Parkinson's).

Some risk factors that can raise homocyseine levels include high alcohol consumption and drinking 8 or more cups of coffee per day. Men tend to have higher homocysteine levels than women, and women's homocyseine levels rise after menopause. Seniors tend to be at greater risk, coinciding with the fact that the elderly most often have significant deficiencies of B6, B12 and folate, which also contribute to a decline in their cognitive function.

Data from such large and respected trials as the *Nurses' Health Study* and *Harvard Physicians' Study* have shown that daily supplementation of these three key dietary vitamins neutralizes high levels of homocysteine. In one placebo-controlled clinical study of 100 men with hyperhomocyteinemia, oral therapy with 650 mcg of folic acid, 400 mcg of vitamin B12 and 10 mg of vitamin B6 in combination was given daily for 6 weeks. At the end of the 6 weeks plasma homocysteine levels were reduced by 49.8%; more about these remedies in Chapter 6 of this book.

C-REACTIVE PROTEINS (CRP)

A multi-billion dollar industry has been built around the concept that large, cholesterol-filled blockages in the arteries cause heart attacks. That concept is plain wrong. The reality is that as many as 80% of all heart attacks occur when smaller plaques, destabilized by inflammation, rupture and attract a blood clot that blocks blood flow to the heart.

So while cardiologists are placing stents to prop open large blockages or bypassing them all together with surgery, inflammation—the real culprit in heart disease—continues unimpeded.

The real culprit is inflammation in the arteries, not cholesterol. In fact, even the *American Heart Association* is now agreeing that people with heart disease all have one factor in common—inflammation in their arteries.

Inflammation is the body's frontline immunological response. Without it you would fall prey to each and every infection that comes along. But sometimes inflammation turns from friend to foe, and that is precisely what is going on in coronary artery disease.

Although there are many markers for inflammation, the best studied for relevance to cardiovascular disease is C-reactive protein (CRP), which is produced by the liver in response to inflammation that occurs within the body. Also, when blood vessels leading to the heart are damaged, the resulting inflammation causes the liver to begin producing this protein. A normal CRP level should be negative to very low, so any elevated reading means there could be trouble. Studies have shown that men with the highest CRP levels have three times the risk of heart attack and twice the risk of strokes as men with the lowest levels. In women, a high CRP level is the single most important predictor of heart attack risk—more so than elevated cholesterol.

This may explain why half of heart attacks occur in individuals with normal cholesterol levels and a quarter occur in people with no risk factors at all. For these clean living folks—who don't smoke, and don't have high blood pressure, high cholesterol, or diabetes—chronic low-grade inflammation and the resulting damage to arteries may be the culprit.

A recent study published in the *New England Journal of Medicine* reported that C-Reactive Protein (CRP) levels could help predict future heart risks, even in people with "low risk" cardiac profiles. In fact, the study showed that high sensitivity-CRP (hs-CRP) was twice as effective as a standard cholesterol test in predicting heart attacks and strokes.

Investigators at the *Brigham & Woman's Hospital* in Boston monitored 28,263 apparently healthy post-menopausal women over a three-year period. In addition to looking at CRP, the researchers evaluated homocysteine and a variety of cholesterol and lipid measurements. Of the 12 markers measured, hs-CRP was the strongest predictor of future cardiac events. We might consider applying the results of this study to men, as well, since CRP has also been identified as a coronary artery disease marker in men.

Inflammation is at the root of the development of plaque in the arterial system and can set the stage for atherosclerosis and provoke cardiovascular events and CRP levels correlate with increased cardiovascular risk. In essence, testing for blood proteins such as CRP can suggest whether or not you have inflamed heart arteries, which can ultimately enhance plaque rupture and lead to a heart attack or stroke.

A new study from the *University of California Davis Medical Center* shows that endothelial dysfunction occurs very early in the atherosclerosis process. What scientists found is that C-reactive protein plays a critical role in atherogenesis by inducing endothelial dysfunction (arterial wall damage). This new finding provides an even stronger reason to test one's blood for C-reactive protein every year. If elevated simple steps can be taken to suppress this destructive inflammatory factor. But the sad truth is few practicing physicians know how to suppress elevated C-reactive protein and most do not even test their patient's blood for it.

If you want to be tested, make sure you ask for the newer, high-sensitivity test called hs-CRP. This CRP test is inexpensive and easy to perform, and should be considered by anyone interested in assessing their cardiovascular risk. Ask your doctor or call your nearest laboratory, whether hospital or off-site lab, and ask if they have the equipment to do hs-CRP tests.

A high level of inflammation is not just an indicator of heart attack and stroke, but research reveals that individuals who have elevated CRP levels are at greater risk of macular degeneration, hypertension, Type 2 diabetes, peripheral artery disease, colon cancer, osteoporosis, and Alzheimer's. In fact, an elevated CRP level is a marker for increased risk of premature death.

Natural remedies to lower CRP include: Low-fat, high-fiber diet, exercise, arginine, omega-3 essential fatty acids, high-dose multivitamin and mineral, curcumin, guggulipid, garlic and ginger; more about these therapies in Chapter 6 of this book.

LIPOPROTEIN(A) OR LP(A)

Lp(a) is a cholesterol particle that causes inflammation and clogging of blood vessels. Actually, it is an LDL particle that has an adhesive protein surrounding it, giving it sticky properties. According to a German physician, Matthias Rath, and other researchers, Lp(a) deposition in arterial walls causes inflammation because of its repair properties.

Under normal circumstances, Lp(a) is one of the most effective repair molecules in your artery walls. In the presence of a vitamin C deficiency, however, Lp(a) can become one of the most dangerous risk factors for artherosclerosis.

Lp(a) has a unique relationship with vitamin C. A key indicator of this relationship is the fact that Lp(a) is found primarily in humans and animal species that are also unable to make their own vitamin C, such as guinea pigs and bats. In fact, animals whose bodies produce optimum amounts of vitamin C (30,000 mg/day) do not have significant amounts of Lp(a) in their blood.

Dr. Rath feels that Lp(a) is a compensatory mechanism in species vulnerable to diminished quantities of vitamin C. In these species, Lp(a) accomplishes blood vessel repair and wound healing. The problem is that while your Lp(a) is running around trying to heal "wounded" or atherosclerotic areas of your body, it simultaneously causes an inflammatory response that can gradually build up puffy little obstructions in your blood vessels.

A recent study published in *Circulation* (a journal published by the *American Heart Association*) showed that this little-known fat particle had an enormous impact on coronary artery disease; in fact, the higher the elevation of Lp(a), the increased risk of heart disease.

Unlike other components of your cholesterol count, the amount of Lp(a) in your blood is not affected by your habits—dietary or otherwise. **Lp(a) is an entirely hereditary factor, so you must change your parents to lower your genetically determined Lp(a) level**.

If you have a family history of heart disease, be sure to have your Lp(a) checked. It could be the missing link in your preventive cardiology program. If your Lp(a) is elevated, take serious measures to reduce it, or at least try to neutralize its inflammatory and clot-promoting characteristics.

There is no known drug that can lower Lp(a) levels. Apparently the pharmaceutical companies have yet to figure out a way to make a fortune treating Lp(a). And research has shown that 34% of patients taking statin drugs (LDL lowering drugs) will bump up their Lp(a) even more.

Natural remedies include: High-dose vitamin C, L-arginine, coenzyme Q10, L-carnitine, omega-3 essential fatty acids and niacin; more about these remedies in Chapter 6 of this book

FIBRINOGEN

Your body produces several compounds that make blood clots, one of the most important of which is *fibrin*. Fibrin is made up of sticky protein fibers, which look a little bit like a tangled spider's web. Fibrin's job is to stick to the blood vessel walls and act like a net, forming a lump or plug that stops the bleeding.

Fibrin is also what determines the viscosity, or thickness of blood throughout your entire circulatory system. Normal fibrin levels will give you normal blood flow.

A high fibrinogen level is an independent risk factor for heart disease, which means that it can indicate an increased risk of heart disease in the absence of any other indicators. By itself, a high fibrinogen level can cause an acute arterial blood clot that can lead to a suddenly fatal heart attack or stroke.

People who are at greatest risk for high fibrinogen levels are smokers, woman who take birth control, and post menopausal women (fibrinogen levels seem to soar in this population). And because fibrinogen levels can be a genetic trait, anyone who has a close relative that has coronary atherosclerosis is at risk.

Next time you have blood work done, ask your doctor to add a fibrinogen assessment to the test. If you are in one of the high-risk groups I just mentioned, but are not scheduled to have blood work done for a while, you might want to request the test as soon as you have time. Fibrinogen levels less than 300 mg/dl are favorable, and anything over 360 mg/dl is considered undesirable.

Natural remedies include: arginine, ginger, nattokinase, garlic, fish oil, ginko biloba, vitamin E and bromelain. Or you can eat one healthy fish meal (mercury free please) each week smothered in garlic; more about these remedies in Chapter 6 of this book.

BACTERIA/VIRUS

Just as we have learned that ulcers are primarily caused by bacteria (H Pylori), we have to be mindful of the impact that bacteria and viruses can have on inflammation and consequently, our heart health, as well.

Most cardiologists understand how crucial periodontal health can be to the prevention of coronary disease. Studies have shown that when multiple microbes are cultured in and around teeth, there is a direct correlation with increased inflammation.

We have also cultured arterial plaque and discovered the presence of a variety of bacteria and viruses. Scientists in Hungary have reported nanobacteria cultured in carotid artery plaque. Cytomegalo virus has been implicated in high rates of inflammation and secondary evolution of C-reactive protein (CRP). Chlamydia pneumonia has also been cultured in plaque. Various spirochetes, worm-like bacterial organisms, have been found to cause high rates of inflammation in cardiac patients, who also exhibited high levels of CRP.

So, based upon voluminous data, microbes including stealth bacteria, viruses, and spirochetes (to name but a few), may very well play a much larger role than we have previously thought in the development of coronary artery disease.

One effective way of warding off the threat of microbes is keep your immune system sharp. When you have chronic inflammation, your immune system weakens. This enables more microbes to grab hold, which adds to your inflammation. It is a vicious cycle that you do not want to get caught up in.

In addition, one of the biggest challenges associated with nanobacteria is that they can change their shape and chemical structure, enabling them to hide from your immune defenses. They develop a calcium coating and turn off surface proteins so your immune system literally cannot see them. That makes them very difficult to treat with antibiotics.

You can promote good oral hygiene and ward off harmful bacteria and viruses by diligently brushing, flossing, and visiting your dentist regularly. L-arginine, CoQ10, arjuna, magnesium, vitamin C, and alpha lipoic acid (ALA) are terrific to strengthen your immune system. More about these in Chapter 6.

CHAPTER FOUR
Available Tests To Measure Heart Disease Risk

You may have gotten to the point in your life where you are asking, "Where is my health going and why am I in this condition I am in?" Or you may be saying, "I feel fine and want to make sure I stay that way."

The fact is, the majority of Americans older than 40 years already have a major health problem. Another disconcerting fact is that the majority of illnesses are sub clinical, meaning they smolder under the surface for many years before they are recognized. Whatever your condition, sickness or apparent health, accurately assessing your current health is the proper place to start on your journey to vibrant health.

Since cardiovascular health is key to health in general--and the lack of it is so common--consequently, we all know someone with heart disease, or we have it ourselves. If you're interested in avoiding or ending personal experience with this disease, I have good news for you: the majority of the causes of cardiovascular disease are in our control.

The first and foundational step in gaining or maintaining cardiovascular health is accurately measuring your current condition. Once that is clearly understood, an effective treatment or preventative plan can be made. In this chapter, we will review the most important factors indicating cardiovascular health or disease, collect the information and grade ourselves.

BLOOD ANALYSIS

Most of us have had our blood drawn to determine our cholesterol level. That number alone, however, is actually quite useless.

There is a huge amount of misinformation about cholesterol, leaving most people thinking it is the grinch who steals youthful vitality. The truth is cholesterol is vital for health and we would all be dead without it.

We get disease if cholesterol is too high or too low. But in the broad range of cholesterol levels from 180 to 240 there is no correlation with heart disease. Below 180 there is increased risk of hemorrhagic stroke, depression, and suicide. Above 240 there is increased risk of cardiovascular disease and ischemic stroke.

Over age 70, elevated cholesterol and cardiovascular events no longer correlate. All told, total serum cholesterol alone is a poor indicator of cardiovascular disease. Half of all heart attack patients have normal total cholesterol levels.

So why are doctors recommending statin drugs for cholesterol levels above 200?

Ask the pharmaceutical companies who sponsor the drug studies and also help determine what normal cholesterol levels are. The upper limit of normal total cholesterol recently went down from 220 to 200, creating "disease" in additional millions of Americans. How convenient that the drug companies just so happen to have the "cure" for that disease!

I want to help you avoid that treatment trap. In fairness, compared to many drugs, most of the statin drugs are some of the safer drugs you might take and actually have the beneficial effects of being powerful antioxidant and anti-inflammatory agents. These beneficial features are likely the reason studies show decreased cardiac deaths when they are used.

Nevertheless, the statin drugs' potential side effects are significant. In some they deplete co-enzyme Q10 (CoQ10) within the liver enough to cause liver enzyme elevations and within the muscles to cause myopathy. Also, and this is not published to my knowledge, but in my and several of my physician colleagues' experiences, statins cause depression or loss of motivation in the majority of patients, probably due to alteration of cholesterol metabolism in the brain. As a result, many of these patients are also on SSRI (selective serotonin reuptake inhibitor) drugs (e.g. Zoloft, Paxil, Prosac).

What is it worth to you to avoid depression and loss of motivation?

There are far safer ways to decrease cardiac deaths and treat abnormal cholesterol levels without risking drug side effects. Despite this, you would be astounded by how many patients would rather take a pill with potential severe side effects than consider changing anything else.

As noted above, total serum cholesterol does not correlate with cardiovascular disease in the range of 180 to 240 but certain fractions of that total cholesterol do correlate. These fractions are HDL and LDL cholesterol. This is why you need a Lipid Profile (also called a Lipid Panel) and not just a total cholesterol when you get your blood drawn.

I have compiled two tables below listing the components of cholesterol (i.e. the Lipid Profile) as well as listing several other markers for cardiovascular health and disease. The first table has the usually quoted normal levels and the second table has ideal levels. Normal levels can change depending upon the levels found in the majority of the population as well as upon what health officials decide is normal. Ideal levels are those, which reflect good health. We want the ideal levels for optimal wellness, not just to be normal.

All of the markers listed in the tables are important. For example, you can have normal HDL/Chol ratio, normal homocysteine, normal fasting glucose, but have ferritin outside the ideal range and have cardiovascular disease as a result. It only takes one rascal to spill the beans.

Cardiovascular Disease Markers:

These are the declared "normal" levels that your doctor will use to tell you whether your various serum/blood levels are "normal" (**NOTE: These levels do NOT necessarily mean healthy levels, rather these will include healthy and many very unhealthy patients**):

"Normal" levels	
Total Cholesterol (mg/dL)	Normal range = It changes with age but quite accurate: = Upper level is 230 + age, Max 300 = Lower level is 115 + age Recommended cholesterol level is a moving target. Recently cardiologists are recommending everyone's level should be below 200 at all ages.
HDL Cholesterol (mg/dL)	Normal range = Males 30-70, Females 35-80
LDL Cholesterol (mg/dL)	Normal range = 60-150 below age 20 = 70-180 age 30-50 = 80-210 above age 50
Triglycerides (mg/dL)	Normal range = It changes with age but quite accurate: = Males upper level is 130 + age, Max 200 = Females lowerlevel is 80 + age, Max 165 = Males/Females lower level is your age
C-Reactive Protein(CRP)	Normal range = Below 10 mg/L (1 mg/dL)
Homocysteine	Normal range = Below 17 micromoles/L
Lipoprotein (a) (Lp a)	Normal range = Below 25 mg/dL
Ferritin (Iron)	Normal range = Males 20-300, Females 15-120 ng/ml Iron overload = Above 400 ng/ml
Fibrinogen	Normal range = Males 180-340, Females 190-420 mg/dL
Blood glucose(8 hr fasting)	Normal = <120 mg/dL Borderline DM = 120-140 mg/dL Diabetic = Above 140 mg/dL (W.H.O. definition)
Insulin (8 hr fasting)	Normal = Below 20 microUnits/ml Borderline DM = 21-25 microUnits/ml Diabetic = Above 25 microUnits/ml
Hemoglobin A1C	Normal range = Below 7.5% of total hemoglobin

The following serum levels are the most IDEAL (i.e. beneficial) levels for cardiovascular (CV) health. Having any ONE of these outside the ideal range can cause or indicate CV disease! These ideal or healthy levels are much tighter than the often-quoted "normal" levels referred to by your doctor. Remember "normal" does NOT necessarily mean "healthy". We want **healthy**, not just **normal**:

"Ideal" levels	
Total Cholesterol*	Ideal Range = 180 to 200 mg/dL if less than age 70 Ideal Range = Up to 300 if older than age 70
HDL Cholesterol	Ideal level = Above 50 mg/dL
LDL Cholesterol	Ideal level = Below 100 mg/dL
HDL % or Ratios	Ideal levels = See table below
Triglycerides(TG)	Ideal level = Below 100 mg/dL
C-Reactive Protein(CRP)	Ideal level = Below 1 mg/L (0.1 mg/dL)
Homocysteine	Ideal level = Below 8.0 micromoles/L
Lipoprotein(a) Lp(a)**	Ideal level = Below 10 mg/dL
Ferritin (Iron)	Ideal range = 20-50 ng/ml (Above 80 is trouble)
Fibrinogen	Ideal range = 150-300 mg/dL
Blood glucose(8 hr fasting)	Ideal range = 60-85 mg/dL Pre-diabetic = 95-110 mg/dL Diabetic = Above 110 mg/dL Hypoglycemic = Below 60 mg/dL Critical levels = Below 40 or Above 450 mg/dL
Insulin (8 hr fasting)	Good level = Below 5 microUnits/ml Best level = 2-3 microUnits/ml High risk Diabetes= Above 10 microUnits/ml
Hemoglobin A1C***	Ideal range = Below 6% of total hemoglobin

*Cholesterol: It is not advisable to have total cholesterol below 150 at any age due to increased risk for internal hemorrhage, depression, and suicide.

Note: A mnemonic to help you remember that LDL is the "BAD" cholesterol: LDL = Low Down Loathsome cholesterol.

Lp(a): LDL + APO(a) = Lp(a). Artery blockage (plaque) is composed of 90-100% Lp(a) NOT of ordinary cholesterol. **Lp(a) is a substitute

for ascorbate (Vitamin C). If you are not getting enough Vitamin C to produce collagen for tissue repair, when your arteries become injured they cannot heal properly. If there is inadequate Vitamin C, the next best way to repair your arterial injuries is make a Lp(a) plaque to cover the injury. Unfortunately the plaques tend to continue to grow. Simply removing plaque without restoring the artery to health is like tearing a scab off a wound. You do not want to remove the scab until after the tissue underneath has started healing. Your body needs sufficient Vitamin C so your arteries can heal. Elevated homocysteine can also play a role here and is detrimental because it causes the binding of Lp(a) to fibrin in very low concentrations thereby encouraging plaque formation in the vessel walls.

***HbA1C (also called glycosylated hemoglobin) correlates well with your average blood sugar over the last 3 months. Tight blood sugar control makes a HUGE difference in complications in diabetics and prediabetics. When A1C levels are elevated above 6.5, for every 1 percent reduction in A1C levels there is a 14% to 40% decrease in diabetes-related complications! Diabetics with A1C levels of 6.5 or lower only need to have the test repeated every six months. Those with higher levels should be tested every two to three months until levels drop to 6.5 or lower, while they make corrections with improved diet and additional diabetes medication. Most diabetics have the disease for 10 years before it is diagnosed, but it has silently been doing damage for all those years.

Cholesterol Cardiac Risk Factors		
Cholesterol/HDL Ratio (i.e. Total Cholesterol divided by HDL):		
Cardiac Risk	Ratio in Males	Ratio in Females
High risk (3X):	9.7 to 23.4	7.2 to 11.0
Above average risk (2X):	5.1 to 9.6	4.5 to 7.1
Average risk:	3.5 to 5.0	3.4 to 4.4
Below average risk (1/2):	1.0 to 3.4	1.0 to 3.3
HDL Percentage: HDL/Cholesterol X 100 (i.e. HDL divided by Total Chol X 100):		
Cardiac Risk	HDL in Males	HDL in Females
High risk (3X):	Below 10%	Below 14%
Above average risk (2X):	10 to 19%	14 to 22%
Average risk:	24% (Range 20 to 29)	26% (Range 23 to 30)
Below average risk (1/2):	Above 29%	Above 30%
LDL/HDL Risk Ratio (i.e. LDL divided by HDL) Male or Female:		
Cardiac Risk	Ratio in Males	Ratio in Females
High risk (3X):	6.4 to 8.0	5.1 to 6.1
Above average risk (2X):	3.7 to 6.3	3.3 to 5.0
Average risk:	1.1 to 3.6	1.6 to 3.2
Below average risk (1/2):	Below 1.1	Below 1.6

Besides obtaining blood work, your doctor has other tests he can order to determine your cardiovascular state including resting EKG, treadmill stress test, CT coronary calcium scoring, echocardiogram, nuclear medicine scans, and coronary angiography. These are useful if you have known or suspected disease; however, as you advance from non-invasive to invasive tests, there are increased risks for the tests themselves. There is a one in one thousand chance of dying from a coronary angiogram. This is an average. In your doctor's hands you may have a much lower risk, but it also could be much higher. These tests must be used wisely.

You obviously need to go to a doctor if you want to get the appropriate blood work and the other procedures listed above. But there is "low tech" and yet very useful evaluations you can do on your own which also help determine your cardiovascular risk.

The "Low-Tech" Cardiovascular Evaluations

Smoking

The first evaluation is a simple question. Have you smoked in the past 20 years? The more you have smoked and the more recent the habit, the more detrimental its effect. Chewing tobacco is also injurious but not nearly as much as smoking.

Systolic Blood Pressure

This is the top number of your blood pressure reading. Above 140 mmHg the risk of cardiovascular disease rises as the blood pressure rises.

Ankle-Arm Index

This is also called Ankle-Brachial Index (ABI) and is the ratio of the ankle systolic blood pressure* divided by the arm systolic blood pressure. A normal index is 1.0 and below 0.9 indicates cardiovascular disease.

I mention this test because you may have heard of it, but be aware that it has limited value. The potential weakness of the test is that it tends to be falsely normal in people with calcifications in their arteries, people with diabetes, pre-diabetes, or those with Vitamin K deficiency. Millions of Americans are pre-diabetic or diabetic and most of them do not even know it. Also, recent studies indicate that significant Vitamin K deficiency is becoming common.

So if the Ankle-Arm Index is normal you must exclude these causes of arterial calcification before you can assume the test is truly normal. If the test is abnormal, you have some degree of cardiovascular disease.

*Ankle pressure is taken with the cuff just above the ankle and the stethoscope listening just below the cuff on the inner side of the ankle immediately behind the anklebone.

Resting Heart Rate

An elevated resting heart rate is a powerful indicator of cardiovascular disease in men (however studies have not shown the correlation in women). Healthy = Below 64 beats/min; Mild risk = 64 to 69 beats/min, Moderate risk = 70 to 75 beats/min, High risk = 76 to 80 beats/min, Above 80 beats/min, the risk is three times normal.

Heart Rate Recovery

This test assesses how quickly your heart rate returns to normal after exercise and is quite useful in determining cardiovascular health. This requires that you can reach 85% of your maximum predicted heart rate (your maximum predicted heart rate is calculated as 220 minus your age). If you currently are not accustomed to that degree of exercise, you should get an exercise program from your doctor or a fitness coach and build up to that level slowly. Once you are able to reach that heart rate, you stop the exercise and measure your heart rate 1 minute later. If the rate drops by 12 or less during that minute the test is abnormal and there is significant risk of cardiovascular disease.

Basal Body Temperature

This is a test of your core body temperature and is a very useful test to determine if your thyroid hormonal system is under active (i.e. hypothyroid).

What does being hypothyroid have to do with cardiovascular disease?

Hypothyroidism causes abnormal lipid metabolism, which results in accelerated cardiovascular disease. Cholesterol and other lipids can become elevated due to diminished function of lipid metabolism enzymes, caused by the lower body temperatures. Many body enzymes are highly temperature dependent, malfunctioning at abnormally low or high temperatures. The more abnormal the temperature; the more malfunctional the enzyme. On a molecular basis, this is why we become listless as our body temperatures go out of the normal range and we die at temperature extremes.

Although the frequency of hypothyroidism has been hotly debated for many decades, I am convinced that hypothyroidism is common and often unrecognized. The official normal range of thyroid blood tests is virtually useless except for obvious hypothyroidism and hyperthyroidism. These blood tests are useful if much tighter normal ranges are used. Additionally, accurate assessments of thyroid function can be obtained with basal body temperatures.

Ideally body temperature is taken immediately upon awakening and while still in bed, but it can be taken during the day at least 15 minutes after eating or drinking and when you have not been exercising. Men and post-menopausal women can take their temperatures on any day but menstruating women have some restrictions. Their temperature fluctuates with their menstrual cycle, lowest at ovulation and highest just before menstrual flow. They can most accurately measure the temperature on the second and third day of the period after the flow begins. Normal temperatures are: Armpit 98.0 +/- 0.2, Oral 98.6 +/- 0.2, and Rectal 99.0 +/- 0.2 degrees Fahrenheit.

Another useful assessment is an exceedingly low-tech question, "Do you tend to be very hot or cold when most others are not"? Characteristically, hypothyroid patients are very "cold blooded" and are cold to their core even when wearing warm clothes. As a corollary, these patients rarely can create any significant sweat. As an aside, two other conditions that can cause low body temperature are adrenal exhaustion and profound hypoglycemia but these diagnoses are usually quite obvious.

Gum Health

Do your gums bleed when you brush your teeth even though you do not have a blood coagulation disorder? If they do, you likely have either have periodontal disease or Vitamin C deficiency or both. Either condition predisposes you to cardiovascular disease.

Waist Size

There are many cardiovascular risk formulas and ratios that use your waist measurement, but one of the simplest is also one of the most accurate: Your waist size in inches should not be greater than one half your height in inches. The greater your abdominal girth relative to your height, the greater your risk of cardiovascular disease.

Insurance companies are good at making money because their actuaries are very knowledgeable in determining risks. Why do you think they insist on knowing your height and waist measurements as part of your insurance physical? Increased abdominal girth is a strong indicator of hyperinsulinemia, pre-diabetes, diabetes, and consequently a useful indicator of cardiovascular disease.

CONCLUSION

In summary, we have reviewed several of the most important indicators of cardiovascular health and disease. As Goethe aptly stated, *"What one knows, one sees."* You now have an understanding of cardiovascular health and disease that few others have. You are equipped to see what most will overlook.

If you passed most or all of these tests with flying colors, congratulations, your risk of cardiovascular disease is very low. If you think you need further testing, then let us review together some of the more popular high-tech testing devices and their cost.

THE "HIGH-TECH" CARDIAC EVALUATIONS

Digital Arterial Pulsewave Analyzer (DPA)

The DPA is a tabletop laser device that through a finger pulse wave can measure a person's blood circulation levels and then assign them a grade from A to G; A being the best score.

With the increased longevity of modern societies and the recognition that arterial stiffness is an independent predictor of cardiovascular risk in selected populations, the factors underlying vascular stiffness have assumed major importance. In particular, there has been interest in the association between stiffness and cardiovascular risk factors, such as diabetes and hypertension. It has become clear that arterial stiffness is not solely determined by structural elements within the blood vessel wall and distending pressure, but that there is also functional regulation by the sympathetic nervous system and endothelial derived nitric oxide. This suggests that functional abnormalities, such as endothelial dysfunction, may underlie some of the large artery stiffening found in individuals with cardiovascular disease and risk factors, and thus may be potentially reversible.

The Digital Arterial Pulsewave Analyzer is quick (under 3 minutes), painless, affordable and a very efficient way to grade your risk for cardiovascular disease by reflecting arterial wall function stiffness, associated with hypertension, arteriosclerosis, artherosclerosis and peripheral circulation problems, as well as, reflecting the risk for heart disease associated with left ventricular ejection insufficiency and heart failure.

This state of the art technology can screen a person for a risk factor of arterial stiffness in its early stages and then be used to monitor the therapeutic response in reversing and improving their cardiovascular grade.

Besigns assigning a grade to your vascular health, it will also reveal the biological age of your arteries. You can be a 40-year-old with 60-year-old arteries or vice-versa.

Don't be fooled by the inexpensive price tag for this test, it is very comprehensive and accurate.

Cost: $20 to $50

Electrocardiogram (EKG or ECG)

The 12 lead electrocardiogram (kardio in German, hence the EKG) measures the electric potential of your heart from 12 different directions. Think of it as your personal cardiology fingerprint: it is consistent through time. But if there is stress, a change, or an injury, your EKG will look different from what is normal for you.

A resting EKG gives us information about the heart's conductive system, including current baseline heart rate and rhythm, and possible heart blocks. Voltage measurements (signal strength) indicate relative chamber sizes. Heart positioning and signs of ischemia (poor oxygen delivery) can also be seen.

A record of your EKG when you are healthy is a good baseline for comparison, but resting EKGs have limitations. It can miss problems that might be more evident when your heart is beating faster.

Cost: $50 to $900

GXT or ETT

Graded Exercise Test (GXT) or Exercise Treadmill Test (EET) measures how your heart is functioning when heart rate and blood pressure are increased during the work of physical exertion. These stress tests give us more information than the EKG test.

If coronary arteries are blocked, then giving the heart a little work to do may reveal a potential problem. Most of you are probably familiar with the image of a person walking on a treadmill, hooked up to an EKG, but a stationary bicycle may also be employed for those who have difficulty walking.

Cost: $50 to $900

Echocardiogram

This non-invasive ultrasound of the heart records specific geographical areas of the beating heart, revealing blood flow patterns, and allowing the doctor to measure wall thickness of the heart's chambers. It can also give a good sense of where your valves may be too loose and leaky, or too tight and restrictive.

Your echocardiogram is recorded on videotape, for doctors to easily view, while still images are printed in a report.

This wonderful tool shows how the heart is functioning as a pump, it provides information on ejection fraction (the percentage of blood that is moving out of your heart), and is an overall good indicator of a person's heart health.

Cost: $500 to $1000

Stress Echocardiogram

This non-invasive test combines exercise with an echocardiogram. An echocardiogram is taken with a person at rest and then compared with an echocardiogram taken immediately following exercise.

This test adds diagnostic benefits of real-time ultrasound images to the interpretation of the stress test EKG, making the exercise assessment more predictive. Blood flow to specific regions of the heart muscle can be inferred from how well the heart wall is moving in that area.

Cost: $500 to $1000

Duplex Doppler Ultrasound

This is a diagnostic imaging technique in which an image of an artery can be formed by bouncing sound waves off the moving blood in the artery and measuring the frequency changes of the echoes. It can be used to diagnose the presence of blood clots or blood flow problems in arteries or veins.

Cost: $500 to $1000

HeartScan

This non-invasive test is used to measure the amount of calcium in your heart vessels, which is believed to be correlated to the amount of plaque. The more plaque you have, the more calcium in your coronary arteries.

The HeartScan uses electron beam computed tomography (EBCT) to detect calcium in the heart and coronary arteries. Observation has led researches to suggest that calcium deposits in the vessel wall could be a marker for atherosclerosis (hardening of the arteries).

In a three year study conducted at the *Harbor UCLA Medical Center,* researchers found EBCT scanning was no better than evaluating the standard risk factors predicting who would have a heart attack.

Cost: $250 to $500

EBCT Scans

The Electron Beam Computed Tomography (EBCT) scan assesses "calcium burden," or the amount of calcium that has accumulated in the arteries. The test is quick and simple.

Essentially, you just lie on a table while the scanner takes CAT-scan pictures of your heart. There are no dyes or any other invasive components. The whole test takes less than 10 minutes. You get a little x-ray exposure, but the benefit clearly outweighs the risk of this minimal radiation dose.

This high-tech, high-frequency radiography procedure detects the presence of calcium in the major coronary arteries of the heart. Now, your heart is not like your teeth and bones—calcium is not supposed to be there, so the optimum calcium "score" is zero. Calcification of heart vessels indicates that oxidative stress is taking a toll, or that there is some process going on in the arterial walls that is causing plaque to calcify and harden. Once the scraggly calcium starts hanging on, the vessel walls get more irritated and more inflamed. And even though being calcified may sound like the plaque is solid and securely attached, nothing could be further from the truth. Any patchy, irritated area of a vessel wall attracts red blood cells and fatty molecules, setting off a cascade of inflammatory responses. One thing is for sure...both hard and soft plaques are unstable. Though hard plaque is a little more predictable, both types of plaque are continuously building up and breaking down. We want to promote the breaking down side of this dynamic process.

When you have an EBCT scan, your calcium score will range as low as 0 to as high as 5000. The lower the score the better. And, though a very low score (or even a 0 score), certainly does not rule out non-calcified, soft plaque in your coronaries, a high score over 1000 provides vital information and predictive value about future cardiac events.

According to the research we have so far, a CS score greater than 1000 means that your risk of having a coronary vascular event is approximately 30% over a two and one-half year period.

Cost: $400 to $500

IMT Analysis Scan

For years cardiologists have used ultra sound techniques (bouncing sound waves off a part of the body to create an image) to get moving, real time pictures of such things as cardiac function. In that light, IMT is now as cutting edge as echocardiography was 25 years ago.

IMT analysis is ultrasound imaging of the carotid artery. The measurements obtained from pictures of these crucial arteries to your brain are expressed as carotid artery intimal medial thickness, or IMT for short. Increased IMT is now considered a reliable risk factor for both stroke and cardiovascular disease.

The identification of soft plaque is one of the newer ways to predict who is at risk for cardiovascular disease, including sudden cardiac death. To give you more details, soft (aka flexible) plaque has a greater tendency to rupture than solid calcified (hard) plaque that is seen on EBCT testing as spoken about earlier. One of the big failures in cardiology is that they can identify hard plaques—and even bypass them—only to have what was a less critical (less than 50% blocked) or soft lesion go on to rupture, causing heart attack, stroke, or sudden cardiac death.

In a scientific statement, the *American Heart Association* concluded that carotid artery B-mode ultrasound imaging is a safe, non-invasive and relatively inexpensive means of assessing subclinical atherosclerosis (blockages that do not present clinical signs and symptoms). The group concluded that for asymptomatic people over the age of 45 years, carefully performed ultrasound examinations with IMT measurement could add substantial information to traditional risk factor assessment.

Cost: $400

HRV Holter Monitor

Electrodes are placed on the chest and a recorder is worn on a shoulder strap or belt, which will record every heartbeat over a 24-hour period. Your heart is not a machine that beats at a fixed rate all the time. It varies from moment to moment with activity, emotions, and so on.

This recorded heart rate variability (HRV) can actually be analyzed with computer software programs. HRV is related to your autonomic nervous system function, and is another way of quantifying factors related to psychological distress. The more your heart rate fluctuates, the lower your risk of sudden death.

According to statistics that have been gathered, poor HRV is a definite risk factor for heart disease.

Event Monitor

An event monitor is a device used by a patient for a 30-day period, to provide an EKG recording of the heart's rhythm. It can be activated when the patient feels chest pain, dizziness or an irregular heartbeat coming on and can be used in the diagnosis of arrhythmias

MRI Scans

MRI uses large magnets and radio-frequency waves to produce pictures of the body's internal structures; no X-ray exposure is involved. This technique obtains information about the heart as it is beating, creating moving images of the heart throughout its pumping cycle.

Your doctor uses the MRI to evaluate the anatomy and function of the structures of the chest, including the heart, lungs, major vessels and pericardium (the outside lining of the heart). It is also used to determine the presence of diseases such as coronary artery disease, pericardial disease, cardiac tumors, heart valve disease, heart muscle disease (cardiomyopathy), and congenital heart disease.

The MRI scan takes about 30 to 75 minutes, depending on the extent of imaging needed.

Cost: $400 to $2000

Angiography

Coronary angiography, also called cardiac catheterization, is a procedure in which contrast material is injected through a catheter to see the size and location of plaque that may have built up in your coronary arteries. Angiography is also used to evaluate heart valves, especially if surgery is being considered.

This invasive procedure is done while you are awake and with the use of a local anesthetic. A fine tube (catheter) is put into a blood vessel and maneuvered into a coronary artery. Once the tube is at the heart, dye is injected through this tube. The heart and blood vessels are then filmed while the heart pumps. The picture that is seen, called an angiogram or arteriogram, will show problems such as a blockage caused by heart disease or other problems. Radiopaque contrast material is injected into the groin area (to access the femoral artery), or the bend in the arm (to access the brachial artery). This procedure usually requires percutaneous insertion of a radiopaque catheter and positioning under fluoroscopic control.

Only use this invasive test after the prior listed noninvasive procedures indicate a definite need. Angiography, or cardiac catheterization evaluates the presence and extent of obstructive coronary artery disease.

Cost: $1200 to $5000

The American Heart Association recommends coronary angiography when:

- Tests, such as the cardiac stress test, suggest severe coronary artery disease, especially if several risk factors are present. A stress test compares your EKG while you rest to your EKG during the time and after your heart has been stressed.
- You have severe symptoms, such as chest pain (angina), at rest or with minimal exertion.
- You have an occupation involving the safety of others (pilots, bus drivers, etc.) and are considered at risk for heart attack.

Coronary angiography may not be recommended when:

- Your health problems make it impossible to have coronary artery bypass surgery, surgery to improve blood flow to your heart muscle, or angioplasty, a procedure which opens up blocked coronary arteries.
- You can control your chest pain and other symptoms with medications or other methods.
- You may not want to have coronary angiography if you do not want to or feel that you cannot quit smoking, because you may not receive the full benefit from subsequent treatment.

CONCLUSION

It is important to note: **you cannot test yourself to safety from having a heart attack or stroke.** Even former President Bill Clinton, who is treated by some of the best doctors in America, needed to undergo heart surgery, and that was immediately after he passed a battery of tests with flying colors.

I strongly urge all of you reading this book to seriously consider having a cardiovascular screening using the new Digital Pulsewave Analyzer, which I addressed at the beginning of this section. I have found it to be the best test for evaluating your risk of heart disease because it is quick, painless, non-invasive, very comprehensive and most importantly, very affordable. Find a certified DPA technician in your area and do not fear the results. Knowing the health of your arteries is your first step to preventing or reversing whatever the test reveals and as you will soon discover in Chapter 6 we will look at natural therapies that will do exactly that!

Now we will explore two strategies to winning the war against heart disease. Later we will look at the natural approach, but for now let us begin by looking at how conventional medicine attacks heart disease.

CHAPTER FIVE
Conventional Medicine's Answer

DRUGS

Americans spend an estimated $28 billion every year on cardiovascular drugs. After a trip to the doctor for a regular checkup, testing might reveal elevated levels of cholesterol or blood pressure levels slightly above normal. Because a doctor's time is limited, the average visit lasting 7 minutes, his easiest form of therapy is to prescribe drugs to counter the symptoms. Drugs will work in treating the symptom, but they do not solve the underlying cause, which created the symptom. And drugs do not come without a heavy price tag.

Every time you take a prescribed drug the body adapts to the drug through what is called the **Bi-Phasic Effect**. For example, there are two main types of heart drugs: beta-blockers and calcium channel blockers, but they both do the same thing, which is inhibit the heart muscle from "pumping too hard." That's the first phase: block the muscle. What happens next is the body's response: it slows down. The body's overall oxygen demands haven't changed, but the drug is preventing those demands from being met. The tissues can't get the oxygen they need for normal cell nutrition, so they stop building and they stop repairing normally, as the body learns that it's not going to be getting any more oxygen from the blood. That's Phase Two. Result: gradual overall loss of strength and tissue breakdown. For example, the pancreas shuts down totally since it no longer senses any sugar in the blood, which would require it to make insulin. The end result of the Bi-Phasic Effect is short-term benefit followed by long-term weakening.

Ever know any people who got healthier or stronger or got completely better while they were taking heart medication?

I like what Dr. Patch Adams said to a room full of doctors he was addressing in the movie Patch Adams, *"Our duty, gentlemen, is not to prolong death, but to greatly improve the quality of life!"* I wonder how many people on five to ten medications feel like their quality of life has been improved?

The other issue with prescription drugs is that these drugs place an incredible burden on the liver and kidneys, organs which have to metabolize, detoxify and then excrete all of these drugs and their byproducts. Most people don't understand that the more drugs you put into your body, the more your system has to metabolize. This places an enormous stress on your body. I call it "pharmacologopia"—too many drugs! People simply do not realize that it is not only the high price tag on the drugs that is costing them, but also their bodies are paying a very high price.

The Oath of Medical Ethics that Hippocrates (Father of Medicine) developed and is heard at medical school graduation ceremonies still today, includes the all important words, **"Above all, do no harm."** If Hippocrates were alive today I wonder what he would have to say about the current medical society's teachings and practices. I wonder too if his wisdom would be respected by the very community which he founded. He died in 377 BC, and although we are daily affected by what he began, few stop to think about how it all started. Hippocrates once taught in 365 A.D., *"The only science of medicine is the intelligent use of nature's only real medicinal remedies…herbs. Let food be your medicine and medicine your food."*

The following is a list of medications, how they help, and their potential side effects. Unlike nutritional therapies, drugs are xenobiotic agents, or substances not found in nature. They alter our own biological systems and, as such, can be termed poisons. The theory behind their use is that they bring about a certain desired effect, which in the case of hypertension, is reduced blood pressure. But, as you will see from the information in this section, they have side effects that may be more dangerous than the disease itself.

Diuretics

(Lasix, Lozol, Demadex, Edecrin, Hydrochlorothiazide (HCZT), Aldactazide, Spironolactone, Thalitone, Triamterene, Moduretic, Dyazide, Bumex)

These drugs are prescribed for hypertension and congestive heart failure. They improve the kidney's normal function causing a flood of excess water and salt to be excreted, which in turn reduces the fluid volume of your blood and gives rapid relief to people with excess fluid. However, the long-term use of diuretics to manage high blood pressure dangerously depletes the body of vital minerals, which are lost with increased urination.

20% of people over 65 years of age take some type of diuretic, and in that age group, diuretics have more adverse side effects than any other prescription drug. In the *Multiple Risk Factor Intervention Trial*, a large, double-blind, placebo-controlled study, the diuretic group had an increase in death rate and an increase in the onset of cardiac arrhythmias, even though their blood pressure was lower than the placebo group.

The most commonly prescribed medications for high blood pressure are thiazide diuretics. These diuretics cause marked losses of potassium, magnesium, and every other mineral, which can cause a lot of problems, including irregular heart rhythms. In addition, thiazide diuretics also elevate the blood cholesterol and triglyceride levels, which could offset some of the benefits from lowering the blood pressure, as this would still increase the risk for heart attack. They also elevate blood uric acid levels and sometimes contribute to gouty arthritis, and may bring about or worsen the diabetic condition, a warning that is clearly listed in drug inserts, which no one ever reads, and is listed in the *Physicians Desk Reference.*

Side effects include abdominal cramping, diarrhea, dizziness upon standing, headache, loss of appetite, low blood pressure, loss of potassium, loss of magnesium, stomach irritation, stomach upset and general weakness. Contact your doctor immediately if you experience dry mouth, weakness, drowsiness, restlessness, confusion, seizures, muscle pains or cramps, nausea or vomiting, and men who remain on diuretics for two years had nearly one in four chance of becoming impotent.

Beta-blockers
(Indeal, Kerlone, Levatol, Lopressor, Sectral, Tenormin, Zebeta, Toprol)

These drugs are prescribed for hypertension, congestive heart failure, coronary heart disease, atrial fibrillation, and angina. They decrease the force and rate of heart contractions and are prescribed for angina and high blood pressure. This category of drugs block the ability of your heart to respond to epinephrine and adrenaline, two hormones that get the heart pounding, the blood pressure soaring, and the body sweating and shaking. These drugs can be beneficial for temporary relief, but most physicians prescribe these drugs for indefinite use and maybe contribute to the epidemic of congestive heart failure in this country.

Because beta-blockers reduce heart function, they can precipitate more severe heart failure in people with already reduced heart function. Even people without heart failure can develop a weakened heart after taking beta-blockers for a long time. People with bronchospastic diseases, such as asthma, should not take beta-blockers. People with impaired kidney function should use with caution as this drug is excreted through the kidneys.

Side effects include congestive heart failure, slow heart rate, tiredness, dizziness, depression, shortness of breath and slow heart rate, wheezing, cold extremities, diarrhea, nausea, dry mouth, gastric pain, constipation, flatulence, digestive disorders including heartburn, itching, and rash.

Calcium-Channel Blockers
(Calan, Isoptin, Verelan, Cardizem, Dilacor, Norvasc, Plendil, Procardia)

These drugs are prescribed for hypertension, arrhythmia, and angina. These drugs work by reducing the entry of calcium into the smooth-muscle cells that encircle our arteries and arterioles. Smooth muscles require calcium to contract, so the less calcium that makes its way inside the cell, the less contraction that takes place, allowing vessels to remain relaxed and dilated.

Calcium is an essential component in a variety of cardiovascular functions. Calcium channel blockers may weaken the heart and possibly increase mortality rates. Research has shown that people on calcium channel blockers experienced 60% increase in heart attacks compared to people taking diuretics or beta-blockers. Another study found that older people who took these drugs developed cancer at twice the rate of other people with hypertension.

Side effects include constipation, dizziness, nausea, headache, low blood pressure, fluid retention, pulmonary edema, fatigue, difficulty breathing, slow heart rate, irregular heartbeat, worsening of congestive heart failure and rash.

Your doctor should monitor you for liver damage while on this class of drug and beware that this drug interferes with carbohydrate metabolism. This drug is not for people whose hearts do not pump well (that is, those with an ejection fraction less than 30%).

ACE Inhibitors
(Accupril, Altace, Capoten, Prinivil, Zestril, Vasotec, Monopril)

These drugs are called angiotensin-converting enzyme or ACE inhibitor and are prescribed for hypertension and congestive heart failure. These drugs reduce blood pressure by blocking the production of a substance called angiotensin that constricts the blood vessels. This has a relaxing effect on the artery walls, allowing them to dilate, thus increasing the available space and reducing the pressure against the artery walls.

ACE inhibitors, however, disturb the body's levels of trace minerals, for example decreasing selenium and zinc levels and increasing copper levels. Long-term use of medications that alter any of your natural body functions is obviously dangerous. Such drugs should be used for immediate intervention only, while you are making the necessary changes for long-term correction of under-lying problems.

These drugs can reduce the number of white blood cells in the body; leaving the body vulnerable to infection and making you feel tired and weak. These drugs can also cause kidney and lung damage, and consequently should be avoided by anyone with lung or kidney problems.

Side effects include dizziness, cough, fatigue, nausea, vomiting, chest pain, low blood pressure, diarrhea, headache, weakness, and dizziness upon standing. People with heart failure may also experience heart attack, angina, abdominal pain, fainting, hypotension, cough, bronchitis, difficulty breathing, pneumonia, rash, and urinary tract infection. The most dangerous side effect of ACE inhibitors is an acute swelling of the face, tongue, lips, vocal cords and extremities. This reaction can be life threatening and medical help should be sought immediately if it occurs.

Anticoagulants
(Coumadin, Heparin, Lovenox, Normiflo, Orgaran)

These drugs are prescribed for atrial fibrillation, mechanical heart valves, and prevention of clot-formation after cardiac surgeries or events. These drugs prevent platelets from sticking together and thus reduce the chance of clot formation.

The most serious risk associated with anticoagulants is hemorrhage of tissue or an organ. Less frequently, this drug destroys skin tissue, resulting in rotting or gangrene. Treatment with anticoagulants may increase the risk that fatty plaque will break away from the artery wall and lodge elsewhere. Immediately report any of the following symptoms to your physician: abdominal pain, abrupt and intense pain in the leg, foot or toes, bluish mottling of the skin on your legs, feet or hands, foot ulcers, high blood pressure, muscle pain, rash, thigh or back pain.

Side effects include fatal or non-fatal hemorrhage symptoms such as: paralysis, pins-and-needles sensation, headache, chest pain, abdomen pain, muscle pain, joint pain, dizziness, shortness of breath, difficulty breathing or swallowing, unexplained swelling, weakness, low blood pressure, and unexplained shock.

Limit your intake of supplemental vitamin E to no more than 200-400 IU per day. And do not take aspirin or ginkgo biloba, which both act as blood thinners.

Coumadin interacts with 75 drugs and other substances, so make sure your go over this drug with your physician before beginning to take it.

Digitalis

(Digoxin)

These drugs are prescribed for congestive heart failure and irregular heartbeat. These drugs make the heartbeat stronger and more efficient, improving circulation. These drugs increase cardiac output, lessening the problems associated with congestive heart failure, such as congestion and fluid retention.

People with kidney disorders require smaller dosages. The use of this drug carries with it the risk of causing fatal heart arrhythmias and failure. People taking this drug should be monitored frequently to ensure correct dosage.

Side effects include change in heartbeat, loss of appetite, vomiting, diarrhea, yellow vision, headache, weakness, dizziness, apathy, and rash.

Anti-Arrythmic
(Tambocor, Cardiquin, Quiniline, Enkaid, Ethmzone, Rhymol, Tonocard, Quinaglute Dura tabs, Quinora, Quinidex extentabs, Mexitil, Norpace, Procan, Pronestyl)

These drugs are prescribed to prevent lethal heart arrhythmias. The major problem with these drugs is their proven safety. When the FDA was questioned about why they approved such an unsafe drug like Tambocor, their excuse was that they had a ***theory*** that these drugs would save the lives of more people by preventing abnormal heartbeats than they would kill by causing abnormal heartbeats. The problem is the FDA had no evidence that these drugs would save even a single life.

A large study conducted by the *National Heart, Lung and Blood Institute* showed that these drugs have killed large numbers of Americans. Even the FDA's own warning in the *Physician's Desk Reference* states that if you take Tambocor, you are twice as likely to suffer a heart attack then if you did not take the drug.

Nitrate & Nitroglycerin
(Isosorbide, Isosorbide Dinitrate, Isosorbide Mononitrate, Nitroglycerin patches, Nitro-Dur Transdermal Infusion, Nitrolingual Pump spray, Nitrostat tablets, and Minitran Transdermal Delivery System)

These drugs are used for coronary artery disease and angina. Chest pain, or angina pectoris, is the body's response to a lack of oxygen to the heart muscle, usually as a result of poor blood supply. These drugs work primarily by increasing nitric oxide, which then relaxes the smooth muscles of the vascular system. This relaxation increases the flow of blood through the heart and around the body. If drug treatment does not control the symptoms and there is evidence of narrow coronary vessels, most doctors will recommend bypass surgery or angioplasty.

The occasional use of these drugs to relieve angina symptoms is very effective; however, studies now show that the regular use of these drugs accelerate atherogenic processes and arterial wall damage (endothelial dysfunction) and cause future cardiovascular events. Thus the regular use of these drugs contributes to the progression of coronary artery disease—the very disorder for which the drugs are being prescribed to alleviate.

These drugs may cause severe low blood pressure, particularly if you are in an upright position. This drug should be discontinued if there is blurring of vision or drying of the mouth. Some people will develop a tolerance to this drug if it is used excessively.

Side effects include headache (possibly severe), vertigo, weakness, palpitations, worsened angina pain, low blood pressure, fainting, rash, and dermatitis.

In Chapter 6, I will reveal a natural alternative to nitroglycerine called arginine, which is completely safe and does not come with these negative side effects. Both the drug and the natural solution (arginine) increase the body's production of nitric oxide, which then relaxes the blood vessels and increases blood flow to the heart, as well as everywhere else in the body.

Statins

(Lipitor, Mevacor, Pravachol, Zocor, Crestor, and Lescol)

These drugs are prescribed for high cholesterol levels. These drugs work by lowering the production of cholesterol in the liver and by altering the way LDL cholesterol enters the cells.

The cholesterol drug industry alone is a 15 billion dollar a year industry giving way to another 37 billion dollars of drugs to treat the negative side effects of the cholesterol drug. Let's take a closer look at cholesterol drugs.

Anti-hyperlipidemic drugs are given to lower cholesterol levels, with the ultimate goal of preventing a heart attack or untimely death from heart disease. Although they may lower cholesterol, they have significant drawbacks, not the least of which is their high price tag, typically $2 per day. Statin drugs are also associated with significant side effects, including liver toxicity, muscle cramps, nausea, constipation, heartburn, hair loss, mental decline, impaired memory, speed up formation of cataracts, and cause fatigue. Further, the *Coronary and Recurrent Event Study*, known as the *C.A.R.E.* study, revealed an unexplainable phenomenon: More women developed breast cancer when taking statins than typically would have in the population-at-large. And there is little evidence that statin drugs reduce the risk of heart attack.

Statin drugs entered the market with great promise in the late 1980's and are wildly prescribed and taken by millions. They replaced a class of pharmaceuticals that lowered cholesterol by preventing its absorption from the gut. These drugs often had immediate and unpleasant side effects, including nausea, indigestion and constipation, and in the typical patient they lowered cholesterol levels only slightly. Patient compliance was low; the benefit did not seem worth the side effects and the potential for use very limited. By contrast, statin drugs had no immediate side effects; they did not cause nausea or indigestion and they were consistently effective, often lowering cholesterol levels by 50 points or more.

During the last 20 years, the industry has mounted an incredible promotional campaign, enlisting scientists, advertising agencies, the media and the medical profession in a blitz that turned the statins into one of the bestselling pharmaceuticals of all time. Sixteen million Americans now take Lipitor, the most popular statin, and drug company officials claim that 36 million Americans are candidates for statin drug therapy.

The "experts" are now saying that no matter how low your cholesterol count, if you are a diabetic then you should take cholesterol-lowering drugs. They are completely ignorant of the well-documented dangers of having too low of a cholesterol level. According to researchers from

Yale University School of Medicine cholesterol levels that are too low are linked to an increased risk of mood disorders, depression, stroke and violent behavior.

What is concerning though is that this is not a lunatic doctor saying this but this advice now is part of the official practice guidelines of the *American College of Physicians*, a major doctors' group which represents more than 100,000 internists. It is difficult for me to understand how this group could get away with such reprehensible misguided recommendations. After I take a few deep breaths though and relax, I understand that any drug company that makes $10 billion a year has access to the most brilliant marketers on the planet and is easily able to influence journals that publish studies that support such nonsense recommendations.

New cholesterol guidelines were issued three years ago that would qualify 36 million people to be on these drugs. Now they want to put the 17 million U.S. diabetics on the drug. Once they get this approved they will clearly push the recommendations to the pre-diabetics, which is another 16 million. So they will be pushing nearly over 65 million people to take their expensive solution. They are making $10 billion on one drug when only 15 million "qualify" to be on this drug, now they will have 65 million "qualifying". Do the math, if they can convince the doctors and the public of this ridiculous recommendation; it means another $30 BILLION in their pockets. And folks that is just for Pfizer, it doesn't include the numbers for the other pharmaceutical companies.

What bedevils the industry is growing reports of side effects that manifest many months after the commencement of therapy; the November 2003 issue of *Smart Money* magazine reports on a 1999 study at *St. Thomas' Hospital* in London (apparently unpublished), which found that 36% of patients on Lipitor's highest dose reported side effects; even at the lowest dose, 10% reported side effects. Let's take some time and look at these side effects.

Muscle Pain and Weakness

The most common side effect is muscle pain and weakness, a condition called rhabdomyolysis, most likely due to the depletion of Co-Q10, a nutrient that supports muscle function. Dr. Beatrice Golomb of San Diego, California is currently conducting a series of studies on statin side effects. The industry insists that only 2 to 3% of patients get muscle aches and cramps, but in one study, Golomb found that 98% of patients taking Lipitor and one-third of the patients taking Mevachor (a lower-dose statin) suffered from muscle problems.

For some, muscle problems show up shortly after treatment begins. In one case, reported in the medical journal *Heart*, a patient developed rhabdomyolysis after a single dose of a statin.

For others, the side effects might not show up for two to three years. A Tahoe City resident developed slurred speech, balance problems and severe fatigue after three years on Lipitor--for two and a half years, he had no side effects at all. It began with restless sleep patterns--twitching and flailing his arms. Loss of balance followed and the beginning of what he calls the "statin shuffle"--a slow, wobbly walk across the room. Fine motor skills suffered next. It took him five minutes to write four words, much of which was illegible. Cognitive function also declined. It was hard to convince his doctors that Lipitor could be the culprit, but when he finally stopped taking it, his coordination and memory improved

From the beginning, statins were known, in very rare cases, to cause kidney failure and even death, as in the case of Baycol. Baycol (cerivastatin) has been linked with 31 deaths in the U.S. (52 total deaths worldwide) and was finally removed from the market by the FDA. Doctors are now recommending that AstraZenica's Crestor be pulled off the market after cases of rhabdomyolysis surfaced in trials of people taking 80-milligram doses.

Active people are much more likely to develop problems from statin use than those who are sedentary. In a study carried out in Austria, only 6 out of 22 athletes with familial hypercholesterolemia were able to endure statin treatment. The others discontinued treatment because of muscle pain.

Neuropathy

Polyneuropathy, also known as peripheral neuropathy, is characterized by weakness, tingling and pain in the hands and feet as well as difficulty walking. Researchers who studied 500,000 residents of Denmark, about 9% of that country's population, found that people who took statins were more likely to develop polyneuropathy. Taking statins for one year raised the risk of nerve damage by about 15%--about one case for every 2,200 patients. For those who took statins for two or more years, the additional risk rose to 26%.

According to the research of Dr. Golomb, nerve problems are a common side effect from statin use; patients who use statins for two or more years are at a 4 to 14-fold increased risk of developing idiopathic polyneuropathy compared to the control group. She reports that in many cases, patients told her they had complained to their doctors about neurological problems, only to be assured that their symptoms could not be related to cholesterol-lowering medications.

The damage is often irreversible. People who take large doses for a long time may be left with permanent nerve damage, even after they stop taking the drug.

Heart Failure

We are currently in the midst of a congestive heart failure epidemic in the United States. While the incidence of heart attack has declined slightly, an increase in the number of heart failure cases has outpaced these gains. Deaths attributed to heart failure more than doubled from 1989 to 1997. Statins were first given pre-market approval in 1987. Interference with production of Co-Q10 by statin drugs is the most likely explanation.

The heart is a muscle and it cannot work when deprived of Co-Q10. Cardiologist Peter Langsjoen studied 20 patients with completely normal heart function. After six months on a low dose of 20 mg of Lipitor a day, two-thirds of the patients had abnormalities in the heart's filling phase, when the muscle fills with blood. According to Langsjoen, this malfunction is due to Co-Q10 depletion.

Without Co-Q10, the cell's mitochondria are inhibited from producing energy, leading to muscle pain and weakness. The heart is especially susceptible because it uses so much energy.

Co-Q10 depletion becomes more and more of a problem as the pharmaceutical industry encourages doctors to lower cholesterol levels in their patients by greater and greater amounts. Fifteen animal studies in six different animal species have documented statin-induced Co-Q10 depletion leading to decreased ATP production, increased injury from heart failure, skeletal muscle injury and increased mortality. Of the nine controlled trials on statin-induced Co-Q10 depletion in humans, eight showed significant Co-Q10 depletion leading to decline in left ventricular function and biochemical imbalances. Yet virtually all patients with heart failure are put on statin drugs, even if their cholesterol is already low.

Of interest is a recent study indicating that patients with chronic heart failure benefit from having high levels of cholesterol rather than low. Researchers in Hull, UK followed 114 heart failure patients for at least 12 months. Survival was 78% at 12 months and 56% at 36 months. They found that for every point of decrease in serum cholesterol, there was a 36% increase in the risk of death within three years.

Dizziness

Dizziness is commonly associated with statin use, possibly due to pressure-lowering effects. One woman reported dizziness one half hour after taking Pravachol. When she stopped taking it, the dizziness cleared up. Blood pressure lowering has been reported with several statins in published studies. According to Dr. Golumb, who notes that dizziness is a common adverse effect, the elderly may be particularly sensitive to a drop in blood pressure.

Cognitive Impairment

The November 2003 issue of *Smart Money* describes the case of Mike Hope, owner of a successful ophthalmologic supply company:

> *"There's an awkward silence when you ask Mike Hope his age He doesn't change the subject or stammer, or make a silly joke about how he stopped counting at 21. He simply doesn't remember. Ten seconds pass. Then 20. Finally an answer comes to him. 'I'm 56,' he says. Close, but not quite. 'I will be 56 this year.' Later, if you happen to ask him about the book he's reading, you'll hit another roadblock. He can't recall the title, the author or the plot."*

Statin use since 1998 has caused his speech and memory to fade. He was forced to close his business and went on Social Security 10 years early. Things improved when he discontinued Lipitor in 2002, but he is far from a complete recovery--he still cannot sustain a conversation. What Lipitor did was turn Mike Hope into an old man when he was in the prime of life.

Cases like Mike's have shown up in medical literature as well. An article in *Pharmacotherapy*, December 2003, for example, reports two cases of cognitive impairment associated with Lipitor and Zocor. Both patients suffered progressive cognitive decline that reversed completely within a month after discontinuation of the statins. A study conducted at the *University of Pittsburgh* showed that patients treated with statins for six months compared poorly with patients on a placebo in solving complex mazes, psychomotor skills and memory tests.

Dr. Golomb has found that 15% of statin patients develop some cognitive side effects. The most harrowing involve global transient amnesia (complete memory loss for a brief or lengthy period) as described by former astronaut Duane Graveline in his book *Lipitor: Thief of Memory*. Sufferers report baffling incidents involving complete loss of memory like: arriving at a store and not remembering why they are there, unable to remember their name or the names of their loved ones or unable to find their way home in the car.

These episodes occur suddenly and disappear just as suddenly. Graveline points out that we are all at risk when the general public is taking statins. How would you like to be in an airplane when your pilot develops statin-induced amnesia?

While the pharmaceutical industry denies that statins can cause amnesia, memory loss has shown up in several statin trials. In a trial involving 2,502 subjects, amnesia occurred in seven receiving Lipitor; amnesia also occurred in two of 742 subjects during comparative trials with other statins. In addition, "abnormal thinking" was reported in four of the 2,502 clinical trial subjects. The total recorded side effects were therefore 0.5%; a figure that likely under-represents the true frequency since memory loss was not specifically studied in these trials.

Cancer

In every study with rodents to date, statins have caused cancer. Why have we not seen such a dramatic correlation in human studies? Because cancer takes a long time to develop and most of the statin trials do not go on longer than two or three years. Still, in one trial, the *CARE* trial, breast cancer rates of those taking a statin went up 1,500%. In the *Heart Protection Study*, non-melanoma skin cancer occurred in 243 patients treated with simvastatin compared with 202 cases in the control group.

Manufacturers of statin drugs have recognized the fact that statins depress the immune system, an effect that can lead to cancer and infectious disease, recommending statin use for inflammatory arthritis and as an immune suppressor for transplant patients.

Pancreatic Rot

The medical literature contains several reports of pancreatitis in patients taking statins. One paper describes the case of a 49-year-old woman who was admitted to the hospital with diarrhea and septic shock one month after beginning treatment with lovastatin.

She died after prolonged hospitalization; the cause of death was necrotizing pancreatitis. Her doctors noted that the patient had no evidence of common risk factors for acute pancreatitis, such as biliary tract disease or alcohol use. "Prescribers of statins (particularly simvastatin and lovastatin) should take into account the possibility of acute pancreatitis in patients who develop abdominal pain within the first weeks of treatment with these drugs," they warned.

Depression

Numerous studies have linked low cholesterol with depression. One of the most recent found that women with low cholesterol are twice as likely to suffer from depression and anxiety. Researchers from *Duke University Medical Center* carried out personality trait measurements on 121 young women aged 18 to 27. They found that 39% of the women with low cholesterol levels scored high on personality traits that signaled proneness to depression, compared to 19% of women with normal or high levels of cholesterol.

In addition, one in three of the women with low cholesterol levels scored high on anxiety indicators, compared to 21% with normal levels. Yet the author of the study, Dr. Edward Suarez, cautioned women with low cholesterol against eating "foods such as cream cakes" to raise cholesterol, warning that these types of food "can cause heart disease." In previous studies on men, Dr. Suarez found that men who lower their cholesterol levels with medication have increased rates of suicide and violent death, leading the researchers to theorize "that low cholesterol levels were causing mood disturbances."

How many elderly statin-takers go through their golden years feeling miserable and depressed, when they should be enjoying their grandchildren and looking back with pride on their accomplishments?

In conclusion, statin drugs should only be considered if you have a history of heart attack, bypass surgery, or angioplasty and you've been unsuccessful at lowering your cholesterol through natural methods or you have coronary artery disease and despite natural methods you continue to have an LDL cholesterol greater than 130 mg/dL (or more importantly, your HDL "good cholesterol" is less than 35 mg/dL). Research shows the risk for coronary heart disease is 2.5 times greater when HDL cholesterol levels fall below 35 mg/dL.

A Washington-based consumer group, *Public Citizen*, began petitioning the *U.S. Food and Drug Administration* to require statin manufacturers to place a severe warning label on the drugs' packaging. In addition, *Public Citizens* wants the FDA to supply a medication guide to be given to all patients filling prescriptions for statins—Lipitor, Zocor, Mevacor, Pravachol, Crestor and Lescol—and to send a letter to all U.S. physicians, warning of the risk of muscle damage with statins.

The bottom line is that treating high cholesterol is one of the absolute easiest things to do in natural medicine. Avoiding grains and sugars, exercising, eating a proper diet and supplementing with arginine is the key to normalizing cholesterol in all but one or two people out of 1,000 who have a genetic problem with LDL receptors. More about this all natural approach in Chapter 6.

Other Cholesterol Drugs

(Colestid and Questran) & (Atromid and Lopid)

The first group of drugs (resins) absorb bile acids from cholesterol in the intestinal tract and cause them to be excreted, lowering cholesterol levels circulating in the blood. Resins have considerable gastrointestinal side effects including constipation, nausea, bloating, and more seriously, reduced absorption of vitamins A, D, E, and K. In the long run, these deficiencies may cause bleeding disorders and vision problems.

The second group of drugs raise HDL levels and lower triglycerides, but they also may cause serious side effects. According to a long-term study published by the *World Health Organization,* Atromid-S actually increased deaths from non-cardiac causes, primarily cancer.

Aspirin

As I am conducting workshops throughout this great country, I am truly amazed at the amount of you that are taking an aspirin a day. I'm sure you are all well aware that at least 103,000 hospitalizations each year are reported from serious gastrointestinal complications from taking aspirins, that aspirin side effects include gastrointestinal upset and bleeding, kidney and liver damage, water and sodium retention and approximately 16,000 deaths each year are attributed to the use of aspirin. But let me clue you in on some of the latest findings on the use of aspirin as a form of prevention for heart attacks.

Antiplatelet agents, such as aspirin, seem to be substantially more effective in reducing the incidence of non-fatal events than in reducing death. Indeed, among large long-term trials after a myocardial infarction (heart attack) **there is no evidence that aspirin saves lives**.

An intervention such as aspirin can reduce non-fatal events in three ways: by genuinely reducing them, by concealing them, or by converting non-fatal events into fatal ones. The failure of aspirin to reduce mortality despite a reduction in non-fatal events in many studies suggests that aspirin may conceal, rather than prevent, vascular events.

Epidemiological data suggest that 25% of non-fatal heart attacks are silent. As aspirin, even at low doses, is an analgesic and because it may provoke dyspepsia (stomach upset), which may create confusion about the cause of chest pain, it is not difficult to believe that aspirin could increase the proportion of silent events from 25 to 30%.

Aspirin increased the risk of sudden cardiac death in every long-term study of heart attacks that reported such events. This increase was from 4.4% on placebo to 5.6% on aspirin in the persantine-aspirin reinfarction (PARIS) study; from 2.0% to 2.7% in the aspirin myocardial infarction study (AMIS); and from 2.0% to 2.4% in the persantine-aspirin reinfarction study (PARIS-II).

This could reflect an increased risk of sudden cardiac death among concealed, and therefore untreated, events. Another possible mechanism by which aspirin may convert non-fatal events into fatal ones is by increasing the risk of hemorrhagic conversion of stroke and heart attacks.

Aspirin could exert a short-term benefit followed by long-term harm, in which case, the benefits and safety of aspirin could be increased by using only a short-term course of therapy. Additionally, aspirin may be harmful in patients with coronary artery disease and heart failure.

Prolonged aspirin use may raise risks for cataracts. Scientists have known that the long-term use of certain drugs, such as corticosteroids, can contribute to cataract development. The investigators found that long-term (more than 10 years) use of aspirin was associated with a 44% higher increase of posterior subcapsular cataracts, compared with nonusers or short-term users of the drug. Posterior subcapsular cataracts are the most common and most disabling form of cataract. This aspirin-related risk was larger among younger (under 65 years of age) individuals compared with older subjects.

People who are taking aspirin in combination with the blood-pressure lowering ACE inhibitor drugs after angioplasty may be at risk for a dangerous drug interaction, according to a study presented at a *American College of Cardiology* meeting. In a study of more than 2,600 people who had undergone an angioplasty--a catheter-based procedure used to clear clogged arteries--the mortality rate was 3.7% in patients on ACE inhibitors and aspirin compared with 1.2% in those on aspirin alone. That's a 3-fold increase in risk of death.

Many believe that, even if aspirin is not effective, it is safe. Aspirin does appear to be relatively safe for the patients included in clinical trials, but as these studies excluded by design patients at risk of adverse events with aspirin and tended to include younger patients with lower multiple morbidity it is likely that aspirin is not as safe as suggested.

Low dose aspirin for cardiovascular prevention may account for more than 30% of all major gastrointestinal bleeding in patients and may also be associated with an increased risk of renal failure.

Finally, there is a widespread view that aspirin is cheap. However, when evaluating the costs of treatment, the amount and type of benefit, as well as the costs of managing adverse effects also need to be evaluated. Very few economic appraisals of aspirin have been done. And further more, there are natural alternatives like arginine, which are extremely safe and can accomplish the same purpose of preventing platelets from sticking, more about these all natural solutions in Chapter 6.

SURGERY

Every year, more than a million Americans submit to angiograms, angioplasties, and bypass surgeries. This unprecedented growth is fueled not by any legitimate need, but by an ever-increasing supply of physicians trained to perform these procedures.

Every month thousands of heart patients hear these terrifying words in their cardiologists' offices: "You are a walking time bomb. Unless we do a catheterization to find the blockages to your heart and do something about them, you could have a fatal heart attack at any time." These terrorizing words lead patients to submit to heart catheterizations, because they assume that this invasive search for heart-artery blockage is necessary to adequately treat their hearts.

Physicians and patients alike are so infatuated with the high technology of heart surgery that its ill effects, even its necessity, are rarely questioned. **The common perception that heart surgery is the only option for most patients with heart disease, that it is medically required, and**

that it saves lives and improves the quality of life is simply not true.
Of course, some people, a small fraction of the 600,000 patients who
have bypass surgery in this country do benefit. However, a plethora
of scientific data demonstrates that for the majority of patients, heart
surgery is not only unnecessary but also dangerous.

To see what is happening here, you must understand the overwhelmingly
powerful financial incentives for doctors to recommend heart surgery.
The heart surgery industry is booming. According to *American Heart
Association* statistics, in 1995 doctors performed 1,460,000 angiograms
(the diagnostic procedure to evaluate the need for surgery) at an average
cost of $10,880 per procedure. This resulted in 573,000 bypass surgeries
at $44,820 each, and 419,000 angioplasties (the balloon procedure for
opening up arteries) at $20,370 each. The total bill for these procedures
is over $50 billion a year. And you can imagine how much these prices
have inflated over the years!

The truth is, there is no scientific justification for the use angiogaphy,
balloon angioplasty and bypass surgery to treat **most** cardiovascular
disease. Now please hear me! When someone's heart cannot be
stabilized medically, symptoms persist, and EKG changes remain,
despite aggressive medical management (i.e., drugs), blood flow to the
heart must be re-established, even if it takes mechanical and invasive
intervention. In other words, when blood flow to the heart muscle
is interrupted abruptly, as it is in an acute heart attack, cardiac cells
become extremely vulnerable to the effects of ischemia (lack of oxygen),
and they start dying immediately, within three or four minutes. We've
learned from research that patients admitted to a coronary care unit with
EKG changes and blood enzyme elevations require a highly aggressive
approach. Acute myocardial infarction (MI) patients, who are treated
quickly with the best invasive procedures we have to date, are more
likely to survive than those treated conservatively. So if I go to the
hospital having a myocardial infarction, I want the best treatment that
money can buy and I want it NOW!

But for most heart disease patients this is not the case and they need
to know the truth about these invasive approaches. Several studies over

the past two decades, involving 6,000 patients with heart disease, have shown that patients funneled into surgical procedures do significantly *worse* than those treated with non-invasive techniques. In fact, one in 25 patients having bypass surgery and one in 65 undergoing angioplasty will die from the procedure.

Traditional medicine approaches heart disease primarily in one of two ways.

Angioplasty

The first is to ream out clogged arteries or flatten deposits in the vessels with an invasive procedure called angioplasty. Every year in this country, about 900,00 angioplasties (the procedure to open up narrowed blood vessels) are performed to treat arteries that have narrowed or are blocked by plaque. If the narrowing is in a heart artery, the procedure involves a balloon catheter (a hollow tube with a small inflatable balloon on its end) inserted through an arm or leg and pushed up to the heart artery. The catheter is placed into the narrow segment so that the balloon is at the site of the blockage. The balloon is inflated and the heart artery is opened up. Over 500,000 are performed each year on the coronary arteries, the rest are performed in the leg, kidney, or other arteries. However, the procedure does come with several risks, which in some cases can be life-threatening.

Any time a doctor threads the catheter up the aorta towards the heart, the catheter may push up against a plaque and break it. This can cause clotting to occur near the plaque. If it happens in the heart artery, it can cause a heart attack. However, if it happens in the aorta artery (this artery feeds blood to the entire body), bits and pieces of plaque and clot can break off and go anywhere in the body.

- In the leg arteries, debris can block the foot arteries causing the toes to become painful and blue, also known as "trash foot syndrome."
- In the kidney arteries, debris can cause kidney failure and a need to go on dialysis.

- In the stomach arteries, debris can cause abdominal pain and even death to the intestines.
- In the neck arteries, debris can result in a stroke.

Angioplasty is an expensive procedure, costing between $5000 and $20,000 depending on, where it is performed, how many vessels are opened, and how many stents are used.

Old school teaching said angioplasty works because the balloon simply compresses the plaque that was narrowing the coronary artery. We now know this view was too simplistic. What actually happens is this: As the balloon inflates, the plaque cracks and the vessel wall tears. The vessel opens up, but it is severely damaged at the site of the balloon inflammation. The endothelium is ripped off the vessel at the site of the angioplasty. This damage causes clotting to occur, which can easily be prevented by giving patients anticoagulant drugs (blood thinners) and anti-platelet drugs at the time of the procedure.

In 1 out of 200 cases, the vessel is immediately obstructed by a clot and the angioplasty fails. When this happens, or when balloon inflation has not sufficiently opened up the vessel, another procedure is used—this time involving a **stent**, a small metal coil that can expand, placed on the site of the obstruction.

The stent is placed over the balloon of the catheter. As before, the catheter is placed into the heart artery and the balloon (covered by the stent) is placed into the narrowed region. The balloon is then inflated, and the stent expands. When the balloon is deflated, the catheter is withdrawn with the stent left behind, holding the vessel open. This technique is successful in 98 to 99% of cases, so it would appear on the surface that this is a very worthwhile procedure, except for one little detail. This procedure brings with it the introduction of a horrible beast known as **restenosis.**

You see the area in the coronary artery, where the stent has been placed, is now injured and your body automatically goes into a repair mode, forming scar tissue made from connective tissue and smooth muscle cells. In some angioplasty patients, the scar formation is excessive, the vessel narrows again, and the chest pain returns. This process of re-narrowing is called restenosis and there is a 40% chance of this happening after the procedure.

Restenosis is an animal unlike any other. Whereas atherosclerosis takes decades to narrow a vessel, restenosis takes a much shorter time—about three to six months and most drugs fail to stop it. Ironically, in an attempt to help blocked arteries through angioplasty, cardiologists often replace atherosclerosis (a disease that can be treated) with restenosis (a disease that is less responsive to standard medical therapy). Recent medical studies have shown that by increasing nitric oxide production in the blood vessels, not only can the plaque be melted away but, restenosis can be averted, more about arginine derived nitric oxide in Chapter 6.

You really have to ask yourself is this procedure worth all the risks? It is also important to remember that angioplasty can reduce the symptoms of heart disease, but not the disease itself. It should be a treatment of last resort. It generally does not save lives, except for those in the middle of a heart attack. If your doctor insists that you need angioplasty for your heart and vessel disease, get a second opinion. Find a cardiologist that believes in non-invasive procedures.

Coronary Artery Bypass Graft

The second approach to heart disease, by traditional medicine, is to cut away the clogged section or sections of the artery and replace it with a new section or sections of arteries grafted from other places in the body. This procedure is called a coronary artery bypass graft, or CABG...known in the medical profession as "cabbage." This is the most frequently performed surgery in the United States at a cost of $50,000 per procedure. The average mortality for CABG surgery is 4% to 10%. And a common side effect to the procedure is cerebral dysfunction—memory loss and mental decline.

According to a study published in the *New England Journal of Medicine*, bypass surgery, compared with less invasive and risky medical therapy, "appears neither to prolong life nor to prevent myocardial infarction (heart attack) in patients who have mild angina (chest pain) or who are asymptomatic (suffer no pain) after infarction in the five-year period after coronary angiography."

In Scotland, a 10-year follow-up of bypass surgery patients found that only 25% remained symptom-free, while 29% had recurrent anginal symptoms, 13% had a repeat bypass or angioplasty, and an alarming 33% died.

A 2001 study done by researchers from *Duke University Medical School* found a high incidence of mental decline in post heart bypass patients. Other researchers have estimated it to be in the range of 33 to 83% of patients. Changes in mental function can occur as a result of physiological changes, from length of time on the heart lung machine (in order to perform bypass surgery the heart must be stopped—you can't sew a graft on a beating heart), postoperative depression, pain relieving medicine, or even worse, messing with the aorta loosens embolic matter (small bits of plaque and blood clots), which can break off, travel up the carotid arteries in the neck, lodge in the blood vessels of the brain, and disrupt oxygen delivery. In fact, according to an editorial in the February 8, 2001, issue of the *New England Journal of Medicine,* 1.5 to 5.2% of bypass patients have a stroke while on the operating table, which results in damage to the brain, sometimes fatal and often permanent.

In conclusion, if you have coronary artery disease but are asymptomatic, or a physician confirms that your angina is very stable, and you have satisfactory quality of life and a normal ejection fraction, then seriously explore other options with your doctor that are less invasive. And if your doctor still insists, then I implore you to get a second opinion. **Always remember, it's your health, it's your choice!**

However, whenever someone with coronary artery disease has an unsatisfactory quality of life, has unstable angina, is at risk of some portion of their heart muscle destroyed by a heart attack, and complimentary medical therapies have been unsuccessful in limiting their symptoms, then invasive procedures may be the only option.

The best ways to prevent heart disease, and even reverse it for that matter, are to place yourself on a program of a healthy diet, exercise, and targeted nutritional supplements. The body is fully capable of healing itself if you give it the proper raw materials, which I am sorry to say are not toxic, poisonous chemicals. Your body can actually produce its own heart medicine, which I am excited to tell you about in the very next chapter.

CHAPTER SIX
Natural Remedies That Work

DIET

One of the primary alternatives to prescription drugs is a healthy diet. Almost all cardiologists and heart surgeons will attest that it is important, but routinely will tell patients that they need an operation first, because "it's too late, diet alone won't work now." This negative bias toward diet is just plain wrong.

Study after study shows that a low-fat diet not only helps prevent heart disease, but actually reverses it. In a study conducted by Dr. Dean Ornish and published in the *Journal of the American Medical Association* (1983), 23 severely ill heart patients were given an extremely low-fat diet, exercise and stress reduction techniques as their major therapy. These patients were having 10 attacks of angina per week! Roughly one-third of them had already had a heart attack, and all of them were taking heart medications. Once they were on the diet regimen, there was a 91% reduction in the frequency of angina. In other words, the attacks were reduced from almost two attacks per day to less than one per week. One year later, this group was compared with another group of heart patients. Not only did the low-fat group experience rapid alleviation of symptoms, but also the diet regimen actually reversed their cholesterol blockages. In comparison, a similar group of heart patients on the standard fare of medications got worse, with progression of blockages in their arteries.

Stay away from the fad diets that call for little or no fat, because your body needs fats for proper functioning—not trans-fats that are found in processed foods, but "healthy" fat from sources like olive oil, nuts, grains (especially flaxseed), and fish.

You'll want to decrease your intake of red meat and organ meats; oils such as safflower, sunflower, and peanut; whole milk, cheese, and yogurt; potatoes, corn, and carrots; rice, breads, cereals (like Corn Flakes), flour-based pastas, bagels, and pastries.

First and foremost, a high-fiber, healthy-fat, Mediterranean-type diet is absolutely essential because you'll get the precious fiber you need to lower your cholesterol (you must get at least 30 grams of fiber each day). On this diet you'll eat plenty of fiber-bearing vegetables and fruits like grapefruit, which contains pectin, an excellent source of fiber.

One pear or apple a day also provides significant fiber. Baked beans, kidney beans, and navy beans also have fiber and, when eaten with oat bran, these foods can lower cholesterol substantially. **Fiber helps prevent the absorption of cholesterol. It soaks cholesterol up into a gelatin-like form, which your body can't absorb.** In fact, research on fiber shows that total cholesterol can be reduced by 11% and LDL cholesterol by 18% over a two to three week period.

Other foods you should increase your intake of include: olive oil, fish and shellfish, tofu, soybeans, tempeh and soymilk, low-fat cottage cheese, feta cheese, grated Parmesan, oatmeal and high-fiber pasta (like spelt), Jerusalem artichoke, asparagus, broccoli, kale, spinach, cabbage, Brussel sprouts, lentils, chick peas, onions, garlic, grapefruit, cherries, peaches, plums, kiwi, rhubarb, pears, apples, cantaloupe, and grapes.

You can also eat chicken and lean meats such as lean beef, turkey, lamb and yes, you can still enjoy the pleasure of occasional desserts. Just be sure not to go overboard with sweets because they can cause secretion of insulin, which may set the stage for heart disease.

EXERCISE

Regular physical exercise raises "good" HDL cholesterol while lowering C-Reactive Proteins. Studies, such as one out of *Emory University,* have shown that even patients who have congestive heart failure due to prior heart damage can exercise. Yet many doctors are terrified to recommend exercise to heart patients. This is somewhat understandable, but severe exercise restriction can be even more dangerous. When heart patients are completely inactive, their condition often worsens.

Exercise will get your blood flowing and keep your arteries and veins elastic and healthy. As your metabolism rises, your liver will create more of the good HDL and clear away the bad LDL. Exercise will help lower your blood pressure by relaxing the muscles of your blood vessel walls and allowing them to expand, and by decreasing the thickness of your blood. Also, induced sweating purges your body of excess sodium.

Physical exertion and emotional stress can be lethal triggers for heart attacks among sedentary cardiac patients who have a history of heart disease. Unlike factors commonly associated with the development of coronary heart disease such as cigarette smoking, lack of exercise, work stress, anxiety and depression, heart attack triggers are very different.

Researchers made an important distinction: exercise reduced the risk of heart attacks for healthy people but had the opposite effect on inactive cardiac patients who might be placing their health in jeopardy by engaging in vigorous activities.

One study revealed that people who seldom exercised were nearly seven times more likely to suffer a heart attack after engaging in strenuous activities over those who exercised more than three times a week.

Experts hope that the findings from this report will prompt physicians to discuss the events leading up to the cardiac event with their patients in order to pinpoint what they were doing hours before the event. The example researchers cited was a patient who suffered a heart attack after enduring vigorous exertion who then became fearful of engaging in exercise in the future. Experts stressed that these patients need to understand that they could still reap great benefits from daily physical activity.

This presents a dilemma among physicians because there are no set guidelines for addressing psychological factors in their cardiac practice. For now, authors of the review made the following recommendations:

- Cardiac specialists should screen for psychosocial issues
- Recognize that some of these issues can be managed within cardiac practice
- Consider referring patients with severe psychological issues to appropriate specialists

There are a number of different health problems that exercise solves:

- High blood pressure
- High Cholesterol
- Stress
- Depression

Exercise Is Your Ticket to Prevent Heart Disease

Even the *American Heart Association* has realized the great importance of the benefits of exercise by adding "lack of exercise" to the list of major risk factors for heart disease.

Research studies have conclusively proven that even in those who live sedentary lifestyles, adding even a moderate amount of exercise to your daily routine reduces your risk of high blood pressure, osteoporosis, breast and colon cancers, depression, anxiety and stress.

However, what concerns me is that most people, especially doctors, don't fully appreciate just how powerful exercise is.

The Exercise Drug

The way I see it: It really helps to view exercise as a drug. The perspective then provides a context of just how powerful exercise truly is in the treatment of serious disease. It also helps one recognize that, like many drugs, the dose needs to be adjusted very carefully. If you are overweight, have high blood pressure, high cholesterol or diabetes then you will want to consider a daily exercise program, working up to 90 minutes per day until you normalize the problem.

Many find walking a useful way to start exercising as it is very low impact and easy on your joints. Walking doesn't require much training and the only equipment needed is a good pair of walking shoes. You can walk just about anywhere and you can do it anytime.

The Problems With Using Walking As a Workout

If you are starting out in poor shape, slow-paced walking will produce benefits. Unfortunately most people will get relatively rapid improvement in their fitness levels after a relatively brief time of walking. Most people will need to increase the intensity of the exercise after a few weeks and walking on a flat surface will simply not cut it for them anymore. If you happen to fall in this group and want to continue walking as your exercise you will need to go indoors on a treadmill and start walking on an incline.

Walking and resistance weight training provide a wonderful balance of cardiovascular and muscle strengthening benefits. Results from a study published in a 1981 supplement to the *International Journal of Obesity* clearly demonstrated that weight loss could reduce elevated blood pressure. In the study, three out of four obese hypertensives attained normal blood pressure with no drug therapy after losing a designated amount of weight.

Exercise regularly, 20 minutes per session, three times a week. Look at exercise as a mood-elevating, longevity-producing experience. Get a buddy to participate in your new exercise regime. It's more fun and it's important to share accountability with each other.

TARGETED SUPPLEMENTATION

Doctors will often tell patients, *"Just eat five servings of fruits and vegetables everyday and you will be getting all the nutrition you need. Don't waste your money on taking vitamins. You just end up with very expensive urine."* The truth is over 60% of doctors now take at least one form of multi-vitamin. In fact, even the *American Medical Association* reversed a long-standing anti-vitamin policy in June of 2002. *The Journal of the American Medical Association* is advising all adults to take at least one multi-vitamin each day. The doctors who wrote the new guidelines stated, *"It now appears that people who get enough vitamins may be able to prevent such common chronic illnesses as cancer, **heart disease** and osteoporosis."*

No heart-strengthening program would be complete without supplements, which should be taken in conjunction with the foods you eat. Supplements provide extra insurance, particularly when you find it difficult to eat all the foods you need to remain healthy.

But please don't just start gulping down pills by the handful, with no real strategy in mind. Your first step should be to **consult with your physician** and let them know you want to try some new, natural supplements. **Never stop taking your prescription drugs,** especially cardiac drugs, on your own! If your doctor gives you a hard time and puts down the information you are providing them with, then **maybe it is time to find another doctor** or healthcare practitioner who does believe in natural therapies and will work closely with you to get your body on course to healing itself. Always remember, **"It's Your Health, It's Your Choice!"** If you would like to find a healthcare practitioner in your local area, try visiting:

- http://www.holisticmedicine.org
- http://www.naturopathic.org
- http://acam.org

Next, don't just run off to the big vitamin chain store. **Not all supplements are of the same quality.** There are a lot of big pharmaceutical companies supplying these big chains with synthetic garbage.

In the last few years, the synthetic vitamin industry shifted gears from a frontal attack to a more seductive deception. They realized that all they had to do was capitalize on the public's exploding desire for better health through nutrition. Indeed, they have capitalized on just two words. The result has channeled billions of dollars into the coffers of the big chemical manufacturers of synthetic vitamins.

The words are **NATURAL and ORGANIC**. The deception is based on letting these words float around and appear on most vitamins sold when actually the FDA has not clearly defined these two words. It is left to the public to assume that these words imply that anything with the words "NATURAL" or "ORGANIC" on them are directly from nature and unadulterated.

This is not true at all as the FDA loosely defines natural and organic as *anything that ultimately comes from nature*. This could be anything under the sun, including chemicals. This means that synthetic vitamins made from coal tars, refined oils and sugar may have the words natural or organic on them. This is an unconscionable criminal act, but it's "legal". It is wrong to put cheap imitations in the place of something truly unadulterated and direct from nature. The people, who believe that they are buying supplemental health as "vitamins", don't know the seriousness of consuming chemicals under the name "vitamins".

The "vitamin" industry is now big business and big business is getting positioned to capture billions of dollars. The following appeared in *USA Today*, December 29, 1998: "Several big pharmaceutical firms entered the dietary supplement business last fall. Among them: Warner-Lambert, Bayer Corporation, and Whitehall Robins Healthcare." The term dietary supplement here means synthetic vitamins, which means laboratory made chemicals.

This conspiracy against public health is two-pronged. It will amass unbelievable profits for the pharmaceutical companies. This vitamin boom is ready to explode. Once big business begins to spend their billions of dollars and gets into the advertising act, as they are beginning to do now, it will then be so big that it will appear as competition to prescription medicine. The pharmaceuticals win either way.

Note the hypocrisy. Whereas, the FDA has muzzled health claims by nutritionists, the floodgates for the same claims by big business are now open. The pharmaceutical companies have seized up a paradigm shift to health awareness and completely reversed it in favor of themselves. They will manufacture worthless placebos by the ton and distribute them as "vitamins" at huge profits. These chemical vitamins will fail as nutrition, as they well know, guaranteeing a return of the masses to prescribed drugs.

Our bodies can cope with starvation better than we can handle chemical toxins under any name. The minute a whole vitamin complex is isolated, it becomes a chemical, not whole food or nutrition. The synergism of the complex is lost.

What you need to do is find a company you can trust. Find a company that manufactures their own supplements in an FDA registered facility, which strictly adheres to FDA Pharmaceutical standards of current Good Manufacturing Practices (cGMP) and does not outsource to a big manufacturer who might alter the formulas to save money on production. Find a company that has been manufacturing for at least ten years, has an impeccable reputation in the supplement industry, does third party batch analysis and can provide a product certificate of analysis upon request. I personally have been buying my supplements from the same company for the last 10 years and am very pleased with the results that, not only I am getting, but also all the people that I recommend their supplements to.

How can you find such a company? Shop around! This is a very important decision and you need to treat it as such. Use the "information highway" known as the Internet. If you do not use the Internet, then ask around. Ask family, friends and work associates if they are taking supplements and how they like them. Remember, everyone has an opinion and are dying to give it to you.

After making a decision, proceed with caution. Try a 30-day supply and record your results with your doctor. Most reputable companies will offer a 30-day money back guarantee. You need to proceed slowly one supplement at a time. How will you know which supplement is working and which supplement is not? Put each supplement through a 30-day rigorous test. Develop a systematic way of taking each supplement and recording the results.

If you are feeling better and/or if the symptoms are improving then you know you got a winner and move on to another supplement. If you do not feel better or the symptoms have not improved, even at the highest dose, then stop taking the supplement, ask for a refund of your money and move on to the next.

It may sound like a lot of extra work, but just how important is your health to you? Would it not be great to never have to take another prescription drug, to never have to fear having a heart attack or stroke or to know with full assurance that you will be around to watch your grand children and great grandchildren grow up? Then you must agree with me, **the results are definitely worth the effort!**

Now, as I have been promising your through this whole book, let us now begin to investigate natural alternatives in supplementation form. I will begin with the one supplement, which I believe to be the most important of all, because it has applications to treat any form of cardiovascular disease including: atherosclerosis, arteriosclerosis, coronary artery disease, peripheral artery disease, carotid artery disease, hypertension, hypercholesterolimia, diabetes, sexual impotence, and restenosis.

ARGININE

***The following information on arginine is the most important information in this entire book. I recommend that you read it over and over until you grasp, with full understanding, the importance of this life saving information, provided by over 69,000 medically published clinical studies on the use of arginine.**

In the book entitled, *"The Arginine Solution,"* doctors Robert Fried, Ph.D. and Woodson Merrell, M.D. stated the following:

> *"In the field of medicine and health it is one of the revolutions of our time: The discovery that the amino acid arginine may be a 'magic bullet' for the cardiovascular system. Now, as the evidence mounts, including research that won the Nobel Prize in Medicine, more and more scientists and doctors see the extraordinary health benefits of increasing arginine intake. A virtual arterial cleanser, arginine helps eliminate blockage and maintain blood flow."*

Arginine is a semi-essential amino acid that has shown promise in the prevention of atherosclerosis. Arginine is the precursor for **endothelium-derived nitric oxide** (EDNO). Three scientists were awarded the Nobel Prize In Medicine in 1998 for discovering nitric oxide's role as a vasodilator (widen the blood vessels). In fact, EDNO is the most potent endogenous vasodilator known. EDNO plays a critical role in the regulation of vascular resistance, as well as in the vasodilation of conduit vessels as they accommodate to increases in blood flow.

In the book entitled, *"The Cardiovascular Cure,"* the author John Cooke, M.D., Ph.D. says this:

"This molecule is nitric oxide, a substance so powerful that it can actually protect you from heart attack and stroke. Best of all, your body can make it on its own. Nitric oxide is your body's own built-in, natural protection against heart disease. We now know that we have a choice regarding this disease. With a diet and lifestyle that channels the natural forces of the blood vessel, atherosclerosis can be prevented, brought to a halt, and even reversed."

Dr. Cooke concludes in his book that the actual 'cardiovascular cure' is a healthy endothelium. When this inner lining of blood vessels is healthy, cells don't stick, clots don't form, arteries don't harden, and you won't die from a heart attack or stroke. It is just that simple!

In the recently released best seller entitled, *"NO More Heart Disease & Stroke,"* the Noble Prize winning scientist Dr. Louis Ignarro says this about arginine derived nitric oxide:

"You do not have to wait for the rest of the world to see the light--and the drug companies to put new Nitric Oxide-based prescription drugs on the market--in order to take advantage of what Nitric Oxide has to offer. Even if you have high blood pressure, have suffered a heart attack, or are at high risk...You can beat the odds. The power to lead an entirely new and healthier life is in your hands. Carpe Diem--Seize the day! Start boosting your Nitric Oxide production right now!"

The Problem

Unfortunately, the problem is there is a long list of conditions that can lower the nitric oxide level in our blood and thus set the stage for an unhealthy endothelium. In fact, the risk factors for atherosclerosis, including high blood pressure, high cholesterol, high homocysteine, alcohol and tobacco use, diabetes, aging, estrogen deficiency, fast foods high in trans fat, and even some prescription medication used to treat many of these conditions, are also associated with low levels of nitric oxide in the blood.

But the good news is **the endothelium can rapidly repair itself** given the right ingredients. Research teams at *Harvard*, *Stanford* and other medical institutions worldwide have carefully documented how within days your endothelium can rapidly recover, simply by increasing the body's nitric oxide production through diet, exercise, and a carefully designed supplementation program.

The Discovery

The most important discovery, about nitric oxide production, came from Dr. Salvador Monacada of England. He announced he had discovered the substance from which endothelium-derived nitric oxide is formed. The substance was an amino acid known as arginine that can be found in protein rich foods, which once ingested, is then converted to nitric oxide.

In fact, medically published clinical studies have proven scientifically that nitric oxide created by arginine will do the following:

- Widen the blood vessels (increasing blood flow throughout the body)
- Soften the blood vessels (reversing the hardening of the arteries)
- Relax the blood vessels (overcoming most high blood pressure)
- Inhibit and melt away plaque (preventing and reversing atheroslcerosis, coronary artery disease, heart attack, stroke and peripheral artery disease)

Dr. Jonathan S. Stamler, a professor of medicine at *Duke University Medical Center*, put it best when he said of Nitric Oxide:

"It does everything, everywhere. You cannot name a major cellular response or physiological effect in which [Nitric Oxide] is not implicated today. It's involved in complex behavioral changes in the brain, airway relaxation, beating of the heart, dilation of blood

vessels, regulation of intestinal movement, function of blood cells, the immune system, even how fingers and arms move."

So the solution is simple...Eat more foods containing arginine! Unfortunately the foods that are richest in arginine are also the foods that a person with an unhealthy endothelium needs to avoid. These foods, like red meat, are also high in fat and cholesterol, big no-nos on your cardiologist's list of foods to stay away from. So what's a person to do? The answer is to get your arginine through oral supplementation Increasing your oral intake of arginine by only 50 to 100% of what you're already receiving from food can begin to impact your health positively in a few short weeks.

In a study done on patients with coronary artery disease, the findings revealed that supplementing with arginine, when used as an adjunct to traditional therapy, improved vascular function, exercise capacity and aspects of quality of life in patients with stable angina within two weeks.

The Proof

Below you will find the essential function and therapeutic effects of arginine. Each health benefit is backed up by scientific research performed by some of the top medical scientists, in the top medical centers around the United States, and published in the most prestigious medical journals. There is at least one clinical study for each of the benefits listed below and can be found in the references located in back of this book.

- Arginine reverses consequences of coronary artery disease
- Arginine improves blood circulation, improves exercise capability and facilitates vasodilation in angina patients
- Arginine helps to prevent atherosclerosis and reduces the severity of existing atherosclerosis
- Arginine inhibits the adhesion of monocytes to the endothelium (an underlying event in the cause of atherosclerosis)
- Arginine improves blood flow

- Arginine helps to prevent abnormal blood clotting (by stimulating the production of plasmin and by increasing vasodilation)
- Arginine reduces blood clots and strokes
- Arginine helps to prevent free radicals-induced damage to the lining of blood vessels
- Arginine improves congestive heart failure
- Arginine significantly increases stroke volume and cardiac output (without effect on heartbeat rate) in congestive heart failure patients
- Arginine increases vasodilation (leading to increased blood circulation) in congestive heart failure patients.
- Arginine decreases high blood pressure.
- Arginine reverses the adverse effects of high blood pressure
- Arginine lowers blood pressure in some hypertension patients (by facilitating the body's production of nitric oxide and by inhibiting the angiotensin converting enzyme (ACE)
- Arginine reduces pulmonary blood pressure and improves blood circulation in pulmonary hypertension patients
- Arginine improves peripheral artery disease
- Arginine improves walking distance in peripheral artery disease
- Arginine increases walking distance in intermittent claudication patients
- Arginine improves outcome after bypass surgery
- Arginine helps prevent restenosis after angioplasty and bypass
- Arginine may give protection against size of heart attack
- Arginine lowers total serum cholesterol levels
- Arginine lowers serum low-density lipoprotein (LDL) levels
- Arginine helps to restore endothelial function in hypercholesterolemia
- Arginine lowers elevated serum triglyceride levels
- Arginine improves diabetes and reverses damage caused by diabetes
- Arginine reduces insulin resistance and improves blood sugar disposal in diabetes mellitus Type 2 patients
- Arginine improves glucose uptake in muscle cells
- Arginine may prevent diabetes

- Argine improves pituitary responsiveness and modulates hormonal control
- Arginine improves asthma
- Arginine increases oxygen uptake in the lungs in persons with hypoxia (due to its role in the production of nitric oxide, which in turn improves blood circulation via vasodilation)
- Arginine improves irritable bowel syndrome
- Arginine improves osteoporosis
- Arginine fights against bacteria, viruses and parasites
- Arginine improves wound healing
- Arginine reduces ulcers
- Arginine improves outcome of cancer treatment
- Arginine improves scleroderma
- Arginine improves alzheimer's
- Arginine improves long-term and short-term memory and cognitive functions
- Arginine improves prostate function
- Arginine improves sexual function, libido, performance and satisfaction in both men and women
- Arinine improves renal (kidney) function
- Arginine alleviates cirrhosis, helps to detoxify the liver, and liver malfunction can occur as a result of arginine deficiency
- Arginine alleviates obesity and facilitates weight loss (by stimulating the release of human growth hormone from the pituitary gland)
- Argine improves muscle performance
- Arginine increases human growth hormone (anti-aging)

The above listed studies are just a drop in the bucket compared to the total amount of clinical studies done on arginine and nitric oxide. In fact, there have been over 69,000 studies dating back to 1927 and they continue to study the effects of arginine derived nitric oxide in the top medical centers around the world.

Safety

Nutritionists have long considered arginine the least toxic of the amino acids, and its consumption, even in relatively huge quantities, seems to have very few adverse side effects. Numerous bodybuilders, for instance, have for years chronically consumed much greater quantities than my recommended dosage, and with no reported ill effects. Moreover, clinical trials at hospitals in the United States and abroad have repeatedly administered 30 to 50 grams of arginine safely to patients, again without reported problems.

Side effects are very rare but may include, stomach upset or diarrhea (taking some carbohydrates with arginine will prevent this).

Arginine is NOT for use by pregnant or lactating women, males with prostate disorders or high PSA values.

Persons under the age of 23 and/or persons who have not completed their long-bone growth phase should not take arginine.

At this time (January-2006) there are no well-known drug interactions with arginine other than people taking nitrate drugs (i.e. nitroglycerine) or vasculogenic drugs (i.e. Viagra), should avoid arginine since blood pressure may drop too low; however, there have been no reports of this adverse event.

The problem regarding ingestion of low-grade arginine formulas is that of the reactivation of herpes and herpes-like symptoms, both oral and genital, which would render a formula impractical for human use. Arginine cannot cause herpes outbreaks, but can exacerbate virus-replication during an outbreak. The herpes virus (herpes virus hominis) typically lays dormant in humans until activated by stress, colds, lack of sleep, and nutritional factors. Low-grade arginine formulas can increase replication of the virus. Lysine is an amino acid that will prevent and help eliminate the herpes virus. Start taking 1000 mg of lysine with 1000 mg of vitamin C at the first sign of an outbreak. Make sure you separate taking arginine and lysine by at least two hours.

Use of arginine is not recommended if you have been diagnosed with cancer. Though arginine has been shown to help successfully combat many cancers, very high doses (30-50 grams of arginine) per day stimulates growth hormone, which primarily stimulates growth of muscle mass. Certain tumor cells **may** thrive on human growth hormone, which **may** stimulate growth of breast cancer cells. As far back as 1981, the *National Cancer Institute* reported that arginine-derived nitric oxide inhibits (blocks) breast-cancer-cell replication in a test tube, and arginine has never been shown to cause breast or any other type of cancer. The research shows the pros and cons of using arginine at high doses. Doses of 6 grams a day or less of arginine is not considered a potential problem for cancer patients, but, as a precautionary decision, use of arginine in the presence of any cancer is not recommended without a doctors specific permission.

What Kind Is Best

Not all arginine is alike and there should be certain things to look out for while perusing the shelves of your local health food store.

First, look for a free-form of arginine, which means the amino acid is in its purest form. Free-form amino acids need no digestion and are absorbed directly into the bloodstream. Also you need to make sure you take between 5 and 6 grams. According to Dr. Louis Ignarro (Nobel Laureate), anything less than 5 grams is a waste of time and money.

Second, look for arginine pyroglutamate. Arginine pyroglutamate is an arginine molecule combined with a pyroglutamate molecule. This is the only free form of arginine that has cognitive enhancing effects and is an excellent growth hormone releaser because it is carried more efficiently across the blood-brain barrier.

Third, read the other ingredients in your arginine formula. Look for other nutrients that will benefit your cardiovascular system. L-citrulline is an amino acid, which will also covert to nitric oxide, but acts as a turbo charger to the arginine's production of nitric oxide. Avoid formulas that contain any other amino acids like: lysine, taurine, carnitine, glutamine, etc. Although these amino acids can also benefit the heart, arginine is the most sensitive of the 22 amino acids and can easily be blocked from absorption by its fellow amino acids. Separate taking any other amino acid supplements or any form of protein for that matter, by two hours before and two hours after taking arginine.

Finally, try to buy your arginine supplement in a liquid form followed by a powder form. Drinking one to four ounces is a lot easier than swallowing 20 to 50 pills and is also much better absorbed. The problem with powders is they take time to fully dissolve and we all know time is one commodity we simply do not have enough of.

"Given such a modest price and all the benefits it can provide to a variety of your bodily systems, medical economists calculating cost-to-benefit ratios would be hard pressed to find a better health-care bargain available anywhere today."

Recommended Dose: 5-6 grams of arginine should be taken daily in a divided dose first thing in the morning and/or last thing before bed. It's best to take with a little carbohydrates to prevent any stomach upset and avoid eating protein at the same time you take the supplement because this may interfere with the absorption of arginine.

Athletes and other fitness enthusiasts will appreciate taking their arginine 45 minutes before a workout or performance, because it is during their workout that the growth hormone is released and this will stimulate the pituitary gland to release more, which translates to an increase in energy, stamina, fat burning and muscle toning.

ARJUNA

Medical science has discovered a remarkable nutrient your heart tissues are craving called, **Terminalia Arjuna (TA)**. Just this one heart-healing nutrient alone has been proven to:

- Boost immunity to bacterial infections

the lead from the men's bodies—an effective cure for lead poisoning. But something else happened to many of the men who were treated with EDTA: they enjoyed an apparent reduction in symptoms of heart disease.

How is this possible? A chelate is a chemical compound in which the central atom (usually a metal ion) is attached to neighboring atoms by at least two bonds in such a way as to form a ring structure. Chelating is the process in which the metal ion reacts with another molecule to form the chelate. EDTA (ethylene diamine tetraacetic acid) is an amino acid. It was synthesized in Germany in 1935, and first patented in the U.S. in 1941.

Chelation therapy itself can be understood simply as the removal of calcium deposits (from your arteries, where you don't want them) and other harmful minerals that promote blood clotting and atherosclerosis. Since these harmful deposits are also known to cause excessive free-radical production, EDTA chelation also functions as a powerful free radical buster, protecting cell membranes, DNA, enzyme systems, and lipoproteins from the destructive effects of these ravenous molecules. Some experts believe that the primary benefits of chelation are due to its free radical-fighting effects. And perhaps one of the most compelling, but often overlooked, explanations for chelation's anti-aging, energizing effects is that EDTA "resuscitates" your cells' mitochondria. Mitochondria are the "power plants" of every cell in the body. Loss of the mitochondria function has long been considered to be one of the primary causes of the aging process.

The *American Heart Association (AHA)* recognizes chelation therapy as a treatment for heavy metal poisoning. The *AHA* admits that EDTA, injected into the blood, will bind the metals and allow them to be removed from the body in the urine. In fact, EDTA is the standard *FDA*-approved treatment for lead, mercury, aluminum and cadmium poisoning. But neither the *FDA* nor the *AMA* acknowledges that **chelation appears to be one of the most powerful, yet least expensive, treatments for heart disease in existence today.** The bottom line: chelation therapy, which costs only $2000 to $4000 per course, represents a significant threat to one of the largest income streams for conventional practioners. Clearly, if EDTA chelation had a large pharmaceutical company advocating its use, it would, at the very least, be integrated into the standard, *AMA*-approved treatment of heart disease. But the patent for EDTA ran out nearly 30 years ago and no patent means no profits. And if the medical industry can't profit from chelation, then this safe, inexpensive, powerful treatment may as well not exist.

From its earliest clinical tests, chelation therapy has consistently demonstrated a remarkable ability to cleanse the system of metals and other deposits that lead to so-called age related disease. In 1955, research conducted at the Providence Hospital in Detroit, Michigan, found that EDTA dissolves "metastatic calcium"—i.e., calcium that has been deposited where it is not wanted: in the arteries, joints, kidneys, and even the bones of the inner ear. In other words, chelation therapy appeared to be a powerful antidote to, and preventive against, atherosclerosis, arthritis, kidney stones, and otosclerosis (hearing loss related to the calcification of the bones in the ear).

In a recent study by clinical cardiologist Efrain Olszewer, M.D., EDTA chelation therapy produced significant results in 2,800 patients. Close to 2,000 of these patients suffered from heart disease and artery disease in the leg, and in this group, there was more than a 90% improvement after therapy. This included significant improvements in the EKG's of heart patients while undergoing stress tests.

Hundreds of papers have been published on the favorable effects of chelation therapy in a variety of chronic diseases. There have been even two massive "meta-analyses" of published and unpublished studies evaluating the results of over 24,000 chelation patients. The results: 88% of the patients demonstrated clinical improvement. In one study, 65 patients on the waiting list for CABG surgery were treated with chelation therapy and the symptoms in 89% improved so much they were able to cancel their surgery. In the same study, of 27 patients scheduled for limb amputation due to poor peripheral circulation, EDTA chelation resulted in saving 24 limbs.

Somewhat less well known, among consumers and health care professionals, are the benefits of the oral form EDTA Chelation therapy, in which the same EDTA compound used intravenously is taken orally, in doses high enough to be effective, yet safe enough to be taken without a doctor's intervention. "It's my firm belief," says Dr. Garry Gordon, MD, DO, "that anyone considering using aspirin for the prevention of heart attack should learn everything they can about oral EDTA. It is my belief that EDTA is as much as 300 times safer than aspirin."

Oral EDTA is not meant to replace IV therapy for those people who have a serious vascular disease.

Recommended Dose: As cited in many studies, dose ranges from 500 milligrams per day to 4000 milligrams per day, with most common doses being around 1000 to 2000 milligrams a day.

NATTOKINASE

This little-known "Japanese Wonder" supports healthy circulation, blood pressure, and overall health.

Japan has one of the lowest disease rates in the world, and one of the best track records for heart health and longevity. No doubt this can be contributed in part to their high fish and seafood consumption. But what's even more intriguing is that they have one of the highest consumption rates of a soybean-based food called natto.

Natto is a fermented food that looks and tastes a bit like cheese. It is made by adding spores of the beneficial bacteria, called *Bacillus natto,* to boiled soybeans. The Japanese have been eating natto for at least 1,000 years, and today the average per capita annual consumption of natto in Japan is roughly 4.5 pounds.

There's a specialized enzyme in natto, called "nattokinase." And it's this enzyme that's emerging as one of the most exciting new breakthroughs for supporting healthy circulation.

Nattokinase was discovered in 1980 by Doctor Hiroyuki Sumi; who at the time was completing his chemistry degree at the *Chicago University Medical School*. He was testing 173 different foods for their ability to promote healthy circulation, and nattokinase did the job better than any of the other substances he was testing.

Since that time, additional research has been done on nattokinase, including 17 published studies in Japan and here in the U.S. The results have been very exciting to say the least. But to fully understand the significance of nattokinase, you need to first understand the impact healthy blood flow has on your entire body.

Normal Blood Flow is the Key to Overall Health

Healthy blood flow affects your circulation, blood pressure and entire body. That's because blood is the transport vehicle that delivers nutrients and oxygen to every cell in your body, carries antibodies where needed, sends the heat in your body out to your skin, and excretes waste products from your body. You cannot be truly healthy without a healthy blood flow.

But here's the challenge. As you age, all of the enzymes in your body may begin to decline—including the enzymes that facilitate healthy blood flow by supporting normal clotting. That's why nattokinase, with its ability to help promote healthy circulation, is such a promising breakthrough.

"Healthy Blood-Clotting 101"

I apologize for getting technical here, but to understand how Nattokinase works, I need to give you a crash course in normal blood clotting. I'll keep it quick and simple.

First off, blood clotting is a normal and necessary process. It is what stops the bleeding if you cut your finger, or suffer from any type of injury.

Your body produces several compounds that make blood clots, one of the most important of which is fibrin. Fibrin is made up of sticky protein fibers, which look a little bit like a tangled spider's web. Fibrin's job is to stick to the blood vessel walls and act like a net, forming a lump or plug that stops the bleeding.

Fibrin is also what determines the viscosity, or thickness, of blood throughout your entire circulatory systems. Normal fibrin levels will give you normal blood flow.

There's Only One Enzyme in the Human Body that Breaks Down Fibrin

While your body makes several compounds that help promote normal blood clotting, it only produces one enzyme-called *plasmin*, which dissolves and breaks down fibrin. Remember, fibrin is what's forming a "web" that stops blood from flowing, so by breaking down fibrin, plasmin helps to keep your blood flowing normally.

Your body produces plasmin all throughout your circulatory system, in the endothelial cells that line the interior walls of arteries, veins, and lymph vessels. But unfortunately, plasmin production often declines with age.

Since plasmin production slows down as you age, it would seem logical that you would want to deliver more plasmin to your body. There is no such thing as a plasmin supplement, but that is where nattokinase comes in.

Nattokinase works to support healthy circulation in two different ways. First of all, nattokinase resembles plasmin, so it can break down fibrin directly. Secondly, nattokinase enhances your body's natural production of plasmin, which also helps to break down fibrin.

In a nutshell, Nattokinase:

- Supports normal circulation, blood flow, and blood viscosity (thickness)
- Supports your body's normal blood-clotting mechanism
- Supports your body's production of plasmin, which reduces fibrin
- Helps to maintain normal blood pressure levels

Nattokinase provides you with support for normal blood clotting, circulation, and normal blood pressure. I recommend taking it right along with your multi-vitamin.

Recommended Dose: 2,000 FU (fibrin units) of nattokinase per day in a divided dose, one nattokinase capsule with your morning meal and another before bed.

D-Ribose

This unique, 5-carbon monosaccharide occurs naturally in all living cells. It forms the carbohydrate portion of DNA and RNA, the very building blocks of life. D-ribose is also a complex sugar that begins the metabolic process for production of adenosine triphosphate (ATP) by your body's 70 trillion cells. ATP is the major source of energy used by the body for normal function. In short, D-ribose is the essential component for your body's basic production of energy. Without D-ribose your cells cannot produce ATP, and without ATP you have no energy. D-ribose is the main fuel that drives the body's cellular engines (the mitochondria), which in turn produces the ATP that gives your body energy.

When the heart does not get enough oxygen, ATP can become depleted. Recent research shows that D-ribose increases ATP production in muscles, including the heart muscle, by between 3.3 and 4.3 times over. According to scientists and doctors, this means that many heart disease patients can greatly benefit from supplemental D-ribose.

One result of poor cardiovascular health is ischemia, a condition where blood flow to and from the heart greatly decreases the amount of oxygen reaching various tissues in the body. When ischemia occurs, the body's cells do not get oxygen to burn energy producing fuels like ATP. Energy levels then plummet, putting more and more stress on the heart, and further reducing energy that would normally be available for everyday life. Medical researchers have demonstrated that during periods of ischemia, ATP levels can plummet by as much as 50% or more. Medical research further demonstrates that even when the ischemia is stabilized, it may take as many as seven to ten days for ATP levels to return to normal. This is why, for many patients with cardiovascular disease, even the simplest activities, required for daily living, may be too difficult. The body is simply not producing the needed energy. This makes energy recovery a major concern for heart disease patients.

But in one study researchers have recently discovered that supplemental D-ribose allows the heart to recover a whopping 85% of its ATP levels within 24 hours! And another study found that, following a heart attack, supplemental D-ribose helped ATP levels and heart function return to normal in just two days. This is absolutely astonishing, considering the fact that without D-ribose, heart function was still depressed after four weeks!

At present, more than 150 peer-reviewed published studies attest to the fact that D-ribose effectively increases ATP while improving performance in heart and muscle cells during periods of lowered blood flow or low oxygen (ischemia). What this means is that supplemental D-ribose can help the heart rebuild energy, and millions of Americans may significantly benefit from its effects.

Research shows that D-ribose can help dramatically improve the quality of life for persons suffering from certain cardiac conditions, and it has a direct positive effect on heart function for persons suffering from ischemia.

D-ribose, being a complex sugar, has none of the unwanted side effects of taking oral ATP supplements and because it goes to work immediately in the body, fueling the mitochondria (the furnace of every cell) so that additional needed ATP is produced for many hours at a time, it works just a s effectively as taking oral ATP.

Recommended dose: Take 5000 mg daily

POLICOSANOL

Policosanol is a compound of fatty alcohols derived primarily from sugar cane or beeswax. And while policosanol is gaining a reputation as a natural alternative to statin drugs, there is more to this supplement than meets the eye; fortunately, most of it is good.

Policosanol is a group of eight to nine 'long-chain alcohols' (solid, waxy compounds). Research is accumulating to show that policosanol is more effective than the most 'popular' (among mainstream doctors) patent medicines for lowering total cholesterol and triglyceride levels.

Policosanol may help prevent strokes by inhibiting platelet aggregation and abnormal blood clotting, and may even lower blood pressure as well.

Even though it is drawn from the same plant that produces table sugar, policosanol does not affect blood sugar levels when ingested. And several studies have shown that it can reduce cholesterol without creating the dangerous side effects associated with statin drugs.

In one trial, reported in the *Journal of Gynecological Endocrinology*, researchers tested more than 240 post-menopausal women with high cholesterol. The subjects were given 5 mg of policosanol daily for 12 weeks, then 10 mg daily for another 12 weeks. After 6 months, researchers found that the supplement was effective in significantly lowering LDL levels (25.2%) and total cholesterol (16.7%). In addition, the women experienced an overall 29.3% increase in HDL level.

Most discussions about cholesterol focus on the ways it endangers the heart. In fact, remember that cholesterol performs several chores that are essential to good health. Cholesterol assists in the absorption of fatty acids, helps manufacture vitamin D, contributes to the production of sex and adrenal hormones, and maintains fatty covers around nerve fibers. As we grow older, however, our hormone levels drop, often boosting cholesterol to levels that cause concern.

One of the common age-related side effects of high cholesterol is a debilitating syndrome of cramping pain in the calves known as intermittent claudication. This is often linked to poor circulation and the presence of arterial fat deposits (atherosclerosis). Removal of those fat deposits, however, has been found to decrease claudication.

Researchers at the *Medical Surgical Research Center* in Havana, Cuba, tested policosanol patients who suffered from moderately severe intermittent claudication. In this two-year study, 56 patients were randomly assigned to receive either policosanol or a placebo. Results indicated that policosanol significantly relieved the effects of intermittent claudication. The 21 people taking policosanol increased their walking distance by at least 50%, while only five members of the placebo group showed a similar improvement.

Other research has shown that elevated cholesterol levels may play a role in the development of Alzheimer's disease, so there is a possibility that policosanol may offer a defense against age-related dementia. This is a controversial topic because much more research needs to be done to determine the exact relationship of cholesterol and Alzheimer's. And yet, we have already seen drug companies subtly (and sometimes not so subtly) promoting statins as a treatment to help prevent Alzheimer's.

Studies have shown policosanol to be generally safe, but there are a few notes of caution.

Of course, a doctor or healthcare professional should be consulted before beginning any new supplement regimen. In the case of policosanol, this is especially necessary for those who are taking blood-thinning medications, or for patients who are currently taking cholesterol-lowering drugs. Also, some study subjects have experienced mild side effects from policosanol, including insomnia, headache, diarrhea, nervousness, and weight loss. These short-term side effects have been reported in less than 1% of the subjects tested. And unlike statin drugs, policosanol has not been shown to have a harmful effect on the liver, the organ that manages the production of cholesterol.

Another concern is policosanol's effect on levels of CoQ10, the antioxidant enzyme that has been shown to promote cardiovascular health, and possibly even help prevent congestive heart failure. One of the ironies of statin drugs is that they have been shown to lower CoQ10 levels. So while you are risking serious long-term side effects to reduce cholesterol, you are also removing a powerful heart healthy antioxidant. Meanwhile, some research has indicated that policosanol may also have a negative effect on CoQ10, although policosanol does not seriously interfere with the body's ability to produce CoQ10.

In any case, a supplement of CoQ10 will be helpful for most people, and some policosanol manufacturers have even added CoQ10 to their supplement formulas.

Recommended Dose: For most people a dose of 5-10 mg per day, but some people need slightly higher doses to lower their cholesterol levels. Naturally, finding the most effective dosage requires careful monitoring of blood tests with the help of a doctor.

This initial monitoring can be problematic; however, because some patients report a rise in cholesterol and triglyceride levels within the first few weeks of policosanol use. Apparently this is not unusual, and in most cases both cholesterol and triglyceride levels can be expected to fall.

ANTIOXIDANTS

Physicians who prescribe cholesterol-lowering drugs rarely recommend taking antioxidants like vitamins C and E or folic acid. This is difficult to understand because these nutritional supplements protect you from free radical damage and have been shown to reduce both fatal and non-fatal heart attacks by as much as 50%, and without the negative side effect.

Free radicals are unstable, electrically charged particles resulting from metabolic processes in your body and dietary and environmental factors. They are extremely toxic to cell membranes, proteins, chromosomes, and DNA. When they attack DNA, they cause mutations that can cause cancer. If free radicals are not contained, they damage everything they touch and start a chain reaction, producing other free radicals until the damage spreads out of control, arterial walls are no longer smooth, and plaque easily accumulates on them. Over time, this clogs arteries and hampers blood flow. By curbing free radicals, you can reverse heart disease and avoid surgery. Antioxidants limit the production of free radicals in your body, neutralize them before they can do damage, and interrupt that damaging chain reaction, which is especially important for protecting cell membranes.

VITAMIN C

Most of us know that blood cholesterol is fractionated into either "good" HDL, or "bad" LDL cholesterol. HDL cholesterol protects against cholesterol blockages, while LDL cholesterol is thought to cause them and is the target of expensive and dangerous heart drugs. But as the late Dr. Linus Pauling showed, LDL cholesterol is not the primary problem. The real culprit seems to be a small particle that resembles LDL cholesterol, Lipoprotein a, or Lp(a), which sticks to small areas of artery damage. They are likened to a small patch that is put on the inside of a bicycle inner tube to repair the tube so the air will not leak out. In this case it repairs small cracks in the artery walls to prevent loss of blood through its walls. After a time, the build up of patches leads to a clogged artery. The problem was not the Lp(a), but instead the original cracking of the artery, which is brought about by the lack of vitamin C in our bodies. Vitamin C is attracted to these damaged artery walls and works to facilitate artery repairs so there is no need for the Lp(a).

Humans, guinea pigs and bats are the only animals in nature that do not produce their own vitamin C. All other animals produce about 30,000 milligrams of vitamin C everyday, and it may surprise you that they do not suffer from heart disease. Vitamin C benefits you in a lot more ways than just preventing scurvy.

Researchers have confirmed Dr. Pauling's thesis. Dr. Ishwarlal Jialal, who won the *American Heart Association's* "Young Investigator Award" in 1989, tested the ability of vitamins C and E and beta carotene to block cholesterol plaquing. Vitamin E was 45% effective, beta-carotene was 90% effective, but vitamin C was a whopping 95% effective.

Recommended Dose: 1000-2000 mg 3 times daily. Note: If you have high iron (ferritin) levels, be careful about mega dosing with vitamin C. Vitamin C enhances the absorption of iron, and too much iron (which can be determined by a blood test) is a risk factor for heart disease.

VITAMIN E

Vitamin E was brought to public notice on June 10, 1946, when *Time Magazine* reported news of "...a startling discovery: a treatment for heart disease...which so far has succeeded against all common forms of ailment...large concentrated doses of vitamin E." Since then, there have been over 6,000 studies on the benefits of vitamin E in the prevention and treatment of cardiovascular disease.

In a study from the *World Health Organization* (WHO), which included thousands of men and women in 16 different countries, a low level of vitamin E in the blood was more than twice as predictive of a heart attack as either an elevated blood cholesterol or elevated blood pressure.

Low levels of vitamin E predicted a heart attack 62% of the time, while elevated blood cholesterol was predictive only 29% of the time, and elevated blood pressure only 25% of the time._

Vitamin E (d-alpha tocopheryl) prevents damage by free radicals formed when fat is exposed to oxygen and heat. Remember it is LDL oxidation, not cholesterol itself that promotes the buildup of plaque in your arteries. When dietary cholesterol has been exposed to heat or oxygen, some of the cholesterol is transformed into extremely toxic particles that irritate the cellular lining of the arteries, initiating the injury that allows cholesterol to adhere to the arterial lining. Vitamin E protects the inside lining of the arteries from these oxidized cholesterol particles.

Recommended Dose: Start with 100-200 IU daily and increase slowly, adding 100 IU each week until daily dosage is 800-1000 IU. If you take an anticoagulant drug, do not exceed 400 IU daily.

BETA CAROTENE

Beta carotene helps protect against heart disease in many ways, the most important of which is its ability to neutralize singlet oxygen, a particle capable of generating and being transformed into more toxic free radicals. Beta carotene absorbs the destructive energy of the singlet oxygen into its own molecular structure and slowly discharges this energy in a safe manner.

Recommended Dose: Daily 10,000-25,000 IUs

OPCs

Oligomeric proanthocyanidins (OPCs) are naturally occurring substances found throughout plant life, however, the two main sources are pine bark extract (Pycnogenol) and grape seed extract. They are unique flavonols that have powerful antioxidant capabilities and excellent bioavailability. Clinical tests suggest that OPCs may be 50 times more potent than vitamin E and 20 times more potent than vitamin C in terms of bioavailable antioxidant activity. In addition to their antioxidant activity, they strengthen and repair connective tissue, including that of the cardiovascular system, as they moderate allergic and inflammatory responses by reducing histamine production. Because they neutralize free radicals, antioxidants are considered nitric oxide's watchdogs, stabilizing and protecting nitric oxide during its brief existence (nitric oxide only has a life span of a couple of seconds)—even extending its life!

Recommended Dose: 100-200 mg daily

POLYPHENOLS

A powerful antioxidant derived from the skin of grapes. In the eyes of science all alcoholic beverages are created equal, however, some drinks may be more equal than others. Red wine may be one of those beverages offering a dual action of alcohol and antioxidants. The name of the game is Red Wine Polyphenols (RWP) - compounds derived from grape tannins and anthocyanin pigments that belong to the most powerful antioxidants in the world. As we absorb polyphenols, they change the properties of blood lipids making LDL-cholesterol more resistant to the sort of oxidation that can trigger atherosclerosis and coronary heart disease.

Recommended Dose: 100-200 mg daily

TUMERIC

The active ingredient in tumeric is curcuminoids, which give tumeric its brilliant color. Tumeric has been shown to lower cholesterol levels significantly faster than pinebark extract or grape seed extract. Curcuminoids not only help to neutralize free radicals, but may actually prevent free radical damage from starting in the first place. Curcuminoids are three times stronger than OPCs.

Recommend Dose: 500 mg daily

CoEnzyme Q10

CoQ10 is a fat soluble, vitamin like substance that is present in every cell of your body. Your cells manufacture CoQ10 naturally, but CoQ10 levels begin to drop as you age.

When your body maintains healthy levels of CoQ10, the risk for cardiovascular disease, as well as a number of other degenerative conditions, may be significantly decreased or avoided. CoQ10 helps prevent premature aging by regulating the use of oxygen in the mitochondria. Every one of the 70 trillion cells, give or take a billion, in your body contain a mitochondria. Here nutrients obtained from the food you eat and the supplements you take are burned in the presence of oxygen. The mitochondria are energy-generating factories, which must have CoQ10 in order to produce energy.

As we age, our bodies produce less CoQ10, which makes them less efficient at absorbing nutrients we take in our food, and while you can get CoQ10 from food sources, it is difficult to get adequate amounts, especially as you age, which is why everyone needs to take it as a daily supplement.

CoQ10 is a key ingredient in any program for healing heart disease. It enhances energy at the cellular level, especially in the heart, enabling the heart muscle to pump blood more efficiently.

CoQ10 is an over-the-counter nutrient that strengthens the heart and is used for angina pain. Most of the research on CoQ10 has been done in Japan, where over 10 million people are taking it on the advice, if not prescription, of their physician.

The heart is one of the few organs in the body to function continuously without resting; therefore, the heart muscle (myocardium) requires the highest level of energetic support. And any condition that causes a decrease in CoQ10 could impair the energetic capacity of the heart, thus leaving the tissues more susceptible to free radical attack.

Studies from around the world have contributed to the mounting evidence that CoQ10 may be effective in treating or preventing cancer, heart disease, muscular dystrophy, Parkinson's disease, periodontal disease, lower high blood pressure, lessen symptoms of Raynaud's disease, relieve allergies, improve stamina in AIDS patients, enhance athletic performance and boost immunity.

Please remember, if you are taking a statin type drug (like I talked about in Chapter 5), then you must add CoQ10 to your daily routine to prevent having muscle pain or a heart attack.

Dietary sources of CoQ10 come mainly from beef heart, pork, chicken livers and fish (especially salmon, mackerel and sardines).

Recommend Dose: For less severe heart ailments 50-200 mg daily, for more severe heart ailments like angina, congestive heart failure or a past heart attack 250-400 mg daily. CoQ10 is best taken with fat to increase bioavailability, so make sure you take it with your meal.

DHEA

It is no secret that most of our serious diseases occur after the age of 50, including heart attacks, cancer, obesity, high blood pressure, diabetes, senility, and Alzheimer's disease. Incredibly, while each problem is associated with its own set of risk factors, a single hormone appears to be universal; low blood levels of DHEA (dihydroepiandrosterone), the "mother of all hormones" is produced by the adrenal glands.

What makes DHEA so unique is that your body converts it upon demand into whatever hormone it needs, such as estrogen, testosterone, progesterone, etc. DHEA is also the only hormone that declines in linear fashion in both sexes.

Elizabeth Barrett-Connor, M.D., from the Department of Community and Family Medicine at the *University of California School of Medicine* in San Diego, tracked DHEA levels in 242 men aged 50 to 79 for 12 years. She found that a 100 microgram per deciliter increase in the DHEA sulfate level was connected with a 36% reduction in mortality from any cause and, in particular, a 48% reduction in cardiovascular disease.

Recommended Dose: 25 mg daily

GARLIC

Researchers continue to amass evidence that garlic contains preventative and healing properties. Research has demonstrated that the sulfur compounds in garlic are the key to its antibiotic and antifungal action, its ability to prevent the liver from generating too much cholesterol, and its tendency to thin the blood and reduce clotting.

During World War II, garlic was known as "Russian penicillin" after the Soviet government turned to garlic after exhausting their supply of antibiotics. Garlic may also have anticancer benefits, in one large study of about 42,000 women, those who consumed garlic in their diet were 30% less likely to develop colon cancer.

A number of double blind, placebo-controlled trials have demonstrated garlic's ability to lower cholesterol and blood pressure and, when combined with onions, fibrinogen levels are also decreased.

Recommended Dose: 500 mg of deodorized garlic twice daily

MAGNESIUM

Magnesium is essential for healthy heart function. It is crucial to produce the high-energy bonds that drive the energy machinery of your cells. More specifically magnesium will:

- **Magnesium reduces blood pressure.** Magnesium is nature's channel blocker. Calcium channel blockers alter the access of calcium into the cell, relaxing the smooth muscle in the artery wall and causing blood pressure to fall. Magnesium functions in much the same way—without dangerous side effects. Numerous studies have shown that supplementation with magnesium often causes a significant drop in blood pressure.

- **Magnesium increases survival of heart attack victims.** A heart attack patient should routinely get intravenous magnesium as soon as he hits the emergency room. Studies show that when a heart attack occurs, there is a massive dumping of magnesium from the heart muscle. This weakens the heart, making it vulnerable to fatal cardiac arrhythmias. Used appropriately, magnesium can be given without toxicity, with amazing survival benefits. In addition, intravenous magnesium can often eliminate cardiac arrythmias when far more dangerous, conventional drugs fail. Dr. Michael Shechter found that magnesium added to the intravenous fluids of patients suffering from a heart attack improved survival by more than 800%! In the magnesium infusion group, there was only one death out of 50 patients, while in the 53 patients receiving a placebo there were nine deaths.

- **Magnesium controls the skipping heart.** Cardiac arrhythmia is a most frightening and dangerous manifestation in patients with heart disease. Given intravenously, magnesium is a powerful stabilizer of heart rhythm. Infusions have been shown to eliminate dangerous cardiac arrhythmias when more routine drugs have failed, and they are exceptionally safe. In a study published in the *Journal of the American Medical Association* (1992), researchers at the *Tufts University School of Medicine* in Boston demonstrated that intravenous infusions of two grams of magnesium to patients undergoing heart surgery dramatically improved their condition. The magnesium-treated patients had significantly decreased cardiac arrhythmia (16% compared to 34% for placebo) and had significantly stronger hearts after surgery as measured by the amount of blood the heart is able to pump. Patients who had very low magnesium levels after surgery had marked difficulty with breathing, and required mechanical assistance with a ventilator much more frequently than patients who had more normal magnesium levels.

- Magnesium helps shuttle potassium and sodium into and out of cells, maintaining proper membrane balance (homeostasis).

Recommended Dose: For men 750-1000 mg daily, in divided doses, after meals and at bedtime.

B-COMPLEX VITAMINS

According to Dr. Kilmer McCully, a Harvard pathologist, most people will be able to keep homocysteine levels under check with supplemental B vitamins and folic acid.

Harvard University tracked more than 80,000 female nurses over a 14-year period and found that a higher intake of folic acid and vitamin B6, exceeding the recommended daily allowance, could help cut the risk of heart disease in half.

Folic acid and B12 are cofactors of methionine synthase, a key enzyme in the homocysteine metabolism. As such, they help to break down the amino acid and convert it into another compound, methionine (which is necessary for proper DNA methylation), indeed pointing to an important role for these nutrients in heart disease prevention. Studies to date have shown that folic acid alone may reduce heart disease risk by as much as 30 to 40%, primarily through its ability to lower homocysteine. However, folic acid works best when teamed up with vitamin B12, which enhances the benefits of folic acid supplementation.

Niacin (B3) is perhaps the most proven supplement for lowering cholesterol and is also the safest. It has been tested in a number of clinical studies and lowers triglycerides as well. Niacin also has the ability to raise HDL while lowering LDL, as well as levels of fibrinogen and LP(a).

Vitamin B1 (Thiamine): A deficiency in thiamine can cause heart palpitations. People who overuse alcohol, have an eating disorder or simply a poor diet, especially one high in carbohydrates, are at higher risk for this deficiency. I recommend taking 50 mg a day, preferably in the morning with breakfast and seeing if your palpitations subside. If they do, you should probably consider re-evaluating your alcohol consumption and diet to solve your problem for good.

Recommended Dose: Folic acid/400 mcg, B6/25 mg, B12/500 mcg, B3/100-300 mg, B1/50 mg.

ESSENTIAL FATTY ACIDS

Omega-3 (alpha-linolenic acid) and omega-6 (linoleic acid) essential fatty acids are vital components of cell membranes, hormones, and nerve cells; and essential fatty acid deficiencies are implicated in many degenerative diseases. They can affect the body's immune system, inflammatory response, blood flow, blood pressure, and coagulability or "thickness" of the blood. Omega-3 fatty acids also can have a marked effect on reducing triglyceride levels. Researchers at the University of Oregon found that 10 patients with markedly high triglyceride levels experienced a drop in triglycerides from 1,353 to 281, and a corresponding drop in their cholesterol level from 373 to 207 in only four weeks on a diet high in fish oils.

The major cardiovascular benefit of increasing fish oils in your diet is not the effect it has on blood fat levels, but on the coagulability of the blood and blood flow characteristics. It is now generally accepted that an abnormal blood clot in a partially blocked artery is a common cause of heart attacks. Fish oil reduces the production of a dangerous substance known as thromboxane A2 that stimulates abnormal blood clots and increases the risk of heart attacks and strokes. In one study of 13 men, 10 capsules of fish oil per day not only reduced the production of the dangerous thromboxane A2, but increased the production of a natural blood thinner, prostaglandin I3.

Two national studies reported, people who eat several servings of fish each week, may lower their risk of heart disease and death.

In one study, men without heart disease were 81% less likely to experience sudden death when their blood levels of omega-3 fatty acids were high regardless of their age, smoking habits, or the amount of other types of fatty acids in their blood.

Omega-3 fatty acids, which are found in fatty fish such as salmon and mackerel, may lower the risk of developing an **irregular heart rhythm** and reduce blood cholesterol and clotting, which are risk factors for heart disease.

The findings point to a way for individuals to lower their risk of **sudden cardiac death** from a heart attack.

The results suggest that increasing intake of omega-3 fatty acids by either supplements or by diet may substantially reduce the risk of sudden death, even among those without a history of heart disease.

More than 50% of people who die suddenly of cardiac causes have no signs or symptoms of heart disease.

In the first study, published in the *New England Journal of Medicine* researchers looked at the experience of about 22,000 male doctors who enrolled in the *Physicians' Health Study* in 1982. They were all free of heart disease at the time, and about 15,000 volunteered a blood sample.

Over the next 17 years, 94 of the men who had given blood samples and who had not subsequently been diagnosed with heart disease died suddenly. The researchers chose about 180 surviving members of the study and compared them with those victims. In particular, they compared the bloodstream concentrations of substances called omega or n-3 fatty acids, found primarily in fish oils.

On average, the men who died suddenly had lower amounts of n-3 fatty acids than the ones who did not. When the researchers divided all the men into four groups based on the concentration of n-3 fatty acids in their blood, the men in the highest quarter had only a fifth the risk of sudden death as those in the lowest quarter.

In the second study, which appears in *JAMA*, researchers studied the experience of 85,000 female nurses. Like the physicians, they volunteered to be questioned and followed over many years as part of the *Nurses' Health Study*, which began in 1976.

The researchers used dietary information gathered in five interviews between 1980 and 1994 to estimate fish intake. They also calculated the approximate amount of n-3 fatty acids consumed, based on the type of fish the women listed in their diet questionnaires.

The researchers found that the more frequently a woman ate fish, the less likely she was to suffer a heart attack or to die of any cardiac cause. Specifically, those who ate fish once a week had a 30% lower risk of heart attack or death as those who never ate fish. Eating fish five times a week was only slightly more beneficial; those women had a 34% lower risk.

Although ocean-living, cold-water oily fish such as salmon, swordfish and tuna offer the largest, easily accessible sources of n-3 fatty acids, there are others. Flax seed oil, canola oil, Perilla oil and English walnuts all contain significant amounts of the oils.

A European study published in 1999 showed that fish oil supplements reduced the risk of sudden death in people who had previously survived a heart attack. The n-3 fatty acids appear to have a specific antiarrhythmic effect, possibly by stabilizing the membranes of heart muscle cells.

The oils also have a blood-thinning effect, like aspirin. In some observational studies, fish consumption has been associated with a lower risk of stroke. There have been anecdotal observations that fish oil supplements may have antidepressant effects as well.

The findings support a growing body of research indicating that omega-3 fatty acids may reduce the risk of heart disease and death.

Almost all fresh, raw, unprocessed nuts, grains, and seeds contain substantial quantities of the omega-6 fatty acids; vegetables and fruits have trace amounts. The flax plant is an abundant source of omega-3 fatty acids. Flaxseeds are 35% oil, 55% of which is an omega-3 fatty acid.

Regularly consuming fish oil and clean, healthy fish is usually one of the strongest recommendations I can advise, as most of you reading this report are dangerously deficient in omega-3s from marine life. However, be warned that fish would be one of the planet's healthiest foods and best sources of Omega fatty acids, except for one very dangerous and sad issue: **nearly ALL fish from ALL sources (ocean, lakes, rivers, & farm-raised) are now highly contaminated by mercury and other toxins.**

Therefore, **I strongly urge you NOT to eat any fish unless you are absolutely certain it has been proven free of dangerous levels of mercury, PCBs, etc.** And be very careful of fish oil supplements as well.

I take an Omega 3-6-9 formulation, which contains exciting new plant oil called Perilla oil that packs a real punch. Perilla is a rich source of omega 3, 6, and 9 fatty acids, phytochemicals and amino acids.

In North America, Zi Su is known by its common botanical name Perilla. Gram for gram, Perilla oil contains more Omega 3 (alpha-linolenic acid) than flaxseed oil. Perilla oil is also a rich source of Omega 6 (linolenic acid) and Omega 9 (oleic acid).

Recommended Dose: 3000 mg of omega 3 and 2000 mg of omega 6 should be divided into three doses daily

CARNITINE

Carnatine is an amino acid which helps convert fatty acids into energy and prevent oxidation stress in mitochondria (powerplants that produce energy for the cells), which can damage the body's cells and ultimately lead to heart disease and neurodegenerative diseases like Alzheimer's.

Studies have shown that when heart patients are given carnitine before an exercise stress test, the heart functions more efficiently: It pumps more blood, with fewer beats, and with less tendency toward oxygen deprivation.

Recommended Dose: Take 2000 mg per day in a divided dose with meals

TAURINE

Taurine is a semi-essential amino acid and a component of bile acids, which the body uses to help absorb fats and fat-soluble vitamins. It is also an antioxidant and in that role helps regulate the heartbeat and maintain cell membrane stability.

Taurine comprises over 50% of the total free amino acids in the heart. It has a positive effect on cardiac tissue and has been shown in some studies not only to lower blood pressure, but also to strengthen the heart muscle, stabilize heart rhythm, and prevent blood clotting.

Because sufficient levels of taurine have been found to prevent brain overactivity and reduce platelet aggression in diabetic patients, this amino acid may someday play a major role in controlling or preventing diabetes, and even Alzheimer's disease.

Recommended Dose: Take 1000 mg per day

SELENIUM

In a study in Denmark of nearly 3,000 people between the ages of 53 and 74, researchers found that those with the lowest levels of selenium in their diets increased their risk of heart disease by 55%. What's more, the researchers suspected that close to 19% of the heart attacks among men in the study might be caused by low levels of this nutrient.

Selenium initiates apoptosis, or cell death, in cancerous and pre-cancerous cells. Cancer cells generally divide rapidly and early. Selenium appears to kill cancer cells before they replicate, thereby short-circuiting the generation of malignancy, tumor growth and cancer spread.

Recommended Dose: Take 70-100 mcg daily

LUTEIN

When news broke a few years back that red wine seemed to protect the French from heart health problems, some of you may have stocked up on Cabernet or Beaujolais. But there's a healthier and less expensive way to protect your heart and your eyes, and that is found in a carotenoid called lutein. This antioxidant nutrient is found in most fruits and vegetables, most abundantly in spinach, kale, and collard greens. Scientists believe that it promotes healthy cholesterol levels and ultimately heart health.

Recommended dose: Take at least 6 mg daily

GINKGO BILOBA

Extracts of the leaves of ginkgo biloba trees have been used therapeutically for centuries in Chinese traditional medicine. Several clinical studies have indicated that ginkgo biloba supplements can improve mental fuctioning in people with Alzheimer's disease.

It is also a benefit for people with poor circulation or peripheral arterial disease (PAD).

Recommended dose: Take 100-300 mg daily

OTHER FORMS OF THERAPY

Doctors are also studying several innovative ways to treat heart disease. Here are a few of the more promising ones.

EECP THERAPY

Enhanced External Counterpulsation (EECP) is an alternative therapy, which was developed by Harry Soroff, M.D., at *Harvard University* 45 years ago as a treatment for angina pectoris, the chest pain associated with heart disease.

EECP dramatically increases the blood flow through the heart arteries, pumping blood from the legs and lower abdomen. It also opens up circulation, making it nature's equivalent to heart bypass surgery. As arteries gradually become blocked, the heart opens avenues of blood around the blockage. By counter-pulsing the blood flow to the heart, the growth of collateral circulation is rapidly accelerated. In no time at all, a whole set of collaterals are opened, supplying adequate oxygen and nutrient-rich blood to the heart muscle and alleviating anginal pain.

In a 1992 study published in the *American Journal of Cardiology*, 18 patients with chronic angina who already had surgery and were being treated with medication were given EECP therapy five times a week. After the full course, 16 of the 18 patients reported complete relief from angina, while the other two had some improvement. Thallium stress tests showed a complete resolution of the obstructive blood flow in 67% of the patients, partial reduction in 11%, and no change in 22%.

The procedure involves the patient lying on a flat or slightly elevated surface, with a body stocking strapped on their lower extremities, from the ankles to just below the waist. The stocking contracts with each beat of the heart, forcing blood up the extremities through the veins back to the heart, increasing blood flow through the body heart muscle and brain. One session lasts about an hour, and there is no discomfort or danger. A usual course is 35 one-hour treatments, given twice a day. In three of four weeks, far less time than it takes to recuperate from a bypass, the problem is eliminated. A full course costs much less than bypass surgery.

TRANSMYOCARDIAL LASER REVASCULARIZATION (TMR)

This procedure improves blood flow to the heart muscle for people with advanced coronary artery disease. Laser beams are used to make channels through the heart muscle to increase blood flow to heart tissue.

ANGIOGENESIS

This involves giving substances through the vein or directly into the heart that trigger the heart to grow new blood vessels to bypass the clogged ones.

CONCLUSION

It is my sincere hope, that this book has helped you to better understand the #1 killer of Americans today. Heart disease is a result of lifestyle factors—high, wrong fat diets, lack of exercise, smoking, heavy drinking, and nutritional deficiencies.

Addressing these deficiencies with natural therapies, which get to the cause of heart disease and not just mask its symptoms, is far more effective at treating and reversing heart disease in the long run than drugs and surgery.

The information and recommendations I make in this book should get you started on the path to preventing or reversing heart disease and achieving optimal health.

Please remember: You must work in close cooperation with your physician and have his or her permission before you begin any drug-lowering program. Although all of the above-mentioned methods are safe, going "cold turkey" on your medication can be very risky. If your doctor does not believe in natural forms of therapy, then I recommend you find one that does. Today more and more doctors are joining the ranks of complimentary medicine.

Remember, wellness is not just the absence of diseases like heart, cardiovascular, or cancer, it is waking up in the morning feeling fresh and alive with vitality. It is having the energy to get through the day without caffeine or other stimulants. It is being physically fit, having good skin, shiny hair, strong teeth, good eyesight and good hearing. It is not having aches and pains. It is having a positive outlook on life.

Wellness depends on a delicate natural balance. In our bodies, doctors call this **'Homeostatis.'** It is the state of equilibrium between various functions. Everything in our bodies is programmed to remain in this balanced state. When your body is out of balance disease and sickness will result. If you can restore the natural balance you will correct the underlying cause for the disease.

Wellness is the natural state of the body. If you make the right **CHOICE** now, all the evidence promises that the quality of life you can enjoy into your sunset years will be rich with both mental and physical pleasures.

Samuel Johnson said, *"To preserve our health is a moral and religious duty, for health is the basis for all social virtues. We can no longer be useful if we are not well."*

Emerson said, *"Health is today, as it has always been, the only form of currency whose presence or absence can make the rich man poor and the poor man rich."*

THE 'KEY' TO GOOD HEALTH LIES WITHIN

Martin Luther's message was simple and clear: neither the church in Rome nor anybody else can sell the key to heaven because the key to heaven is within yourself. This simple message released a storm wind of spiritual liberation. Suddenly millions of people realized that they had been cheated and abused for decades and for one purpose only: the boundless enrichment of Rome.

The storm of liberation was so powerful that the existing systems of the world came tumbling down. On April 18th, 1521, only four years later, Luther was called in front of the emperor's Deity in the city of Worms. In the presence of Emperor Charles V and the pontifical legates, he was pressed to recant in order to stabilize the antiquated order of things. Luther did not recant.

This day in Worms is considered the single most important day in the past 1000 years, because, like no other, it influenced the further development of that millennium. The liberation of the human mind from a century-old yoke of spiritual slavery had become irreversible. Millions of illiterate farmers learned to read and write with the help of the German translation of the Bible. During the course of the 16th century the illiteracy rate in Europe dropped from 80% to 20%. Commerce and trade began to blossom because now people could read and write.

Ulrich von Hutten, a contemporary of Luther, described the incredible feeling of liberation with the words, **"What a joy it is to live."** The medieval times had ended once and for all and the liberation of the human spirit and intellect released resources in all sectors of society and made Europe the most influential continent on Planet Earth.

Today, almost 500 years later, we find ourselves in a similar dependency. This time it is not the dependency of the mind and the intellect, but the dependency of our bodies and our health. Just as it happened 500 years ago, today millions of people are being deprived of their last money for an illusion: health through the pharmaceutical industry.

It is high time that this illusion is ended. Thus, as it was 500 years ago, the message today is simple. **Nobody except yourself owns the key to your health**. The liberation of mankind towards health will liberate similar resources in all sectors of society, like the intellectual liberation 500 years ago.

It is choice not chance, that determines our wellness and our destiny!

REFERENCES

Introduction

Zaret B, Moser M, Cohen l. "What Can Go Wrong?" *Yale University Heart Book,* Hearst Books 1992; 2:12, 3:23.

Karpman H. "The Ticking Time Bomb." *Preventing Silent Heart Disease,* Crown 1989; 1:1-6.

American Heart Association. *Heart Disease and Stroke Statiistics 2003,* Update 2003.

Chapter 1

Williams D. "Taking Aim At Public Enemy Number One." *Alternatives,* Dec 2001; P 42.

American Heart Association. *Heart Disease and Stroke Statiistics 2003,* Update 2003.

Null G. "Types of Heart Disease." *Natural Healing,* Kensington 2001, P. 205-206.

Zaret B, Moser M, Cohen I. "Heart Attacks and Coronary Artery Disease." *Yale University Heart Book,* Hearst Books 1992; 11: 133-135.

Karpman H. "Sudden Death: The Silent Killer Stalks." *Preventing Silent Heart Disease,* Crown 1989; 4: 24-29.

Sinatra S. "Hormone Replacement and Women's Hearts." *The Sinatra Health Report,* Nov 2001, P. 5-7.

Chapter 2

Zaret B, Moser M, Cohen I. "What is High Blood Pressure?" *Yale University Heart Book,* Hearst Books, 1992; 12: 149-156.

Appel LJ. "A Clinical Trial of the Effects of Dietary Patterns On Blood Pressure." *N Engl J Med* 1997; 336: 1117-1124.

Sacks FM. "Effects On Blood Pressure of Reduced Dietary Sodium and the Dietary Approaches To Stop Hypertension (DASH) Diet." *N Engl J Med* 2001; 344(1): 3-10.

Houston MC. "The Role of Vascular Biology, Nutraceuticals in the Prevention and Treatment of Hypertension." *Jana* 2000, Suppl 1:5-71.

Sinatra S. "Lowering Blood Pressure Naturally." *The Sinatra Health Report*, Jan 2002, P. 2-5.

Frohlich E, Subak-Sharpe G. "Exercise and Your Heart." *Take Heart,* Crown 1190, 8: 133-144.

Weil A. "Syndrome X: New Cures For Heart Disease." *Self Healing,* Apr 2001, P. 2-3.

Prevention. "High Blood Pressure: Nix the Drinks." *Healing With Vitamins,* Rodale 1996, P. 299

Siani A, Pagano E, Iacone R. "Blood Pressure and Metabolic Changes During Dietary L-arginine Supplementation in Humans." *Am J Hypertens* 2000; 13(5 Pt 1): 547-551.

Siagy CA. "A Meta-Analysis of the Effect of Garlic on Blood Pressure." *J Hypertens* 1994; 12(4): 463-468.

Fard, A. "Acute Elevations Of Plasma Asymmetric Dimethylarginine and Impaired Edothelial Function In Response To A High-Fat Meal

In Patients With Type 2 Diabetes." *Arterioscler Thromb Vasc Biol* 2000; 20(9): 2039-2044.

Timimi FK. "Vitamin C Improves Endothelium-Dependent Vasodilation In Potients With Insulin-Dependent Dibetes Mellitus." *J Am Coll Cardiol* 1998; 31(3): 552-557.

Abram AS. "The Effects of Chromium Supplementation On serum Glucose and Lipids in Patients With and Without Non-Insulin Dependent Diabetes." *Metabolism* 1992; 41(7): 768-771.

Anderson RA. "Chromium Supplementation of Human Subjects: Effects On Glucose, Insulin and Lipid Variables." *Metabolism* 1993; 32(9): 894-899.

Anderson RA. "Elevated Intakes of Supplemental Chromium Improves Glucose and Insulin Variables In Individuals With Type 2 Diabetes." *Diabetes* 1997; 46(11): 1786-1791.

Mertz W. "Chromium In Human Nutrition: A Review." *J Nutr* 1993; 123(4): 626-633.

McVeigh GE. "Fish Oil Improves Arterial compliance In Non-Insulin-Dependent Diabetes Mellitus." *J Clin Invest* 1994; 92: 105-113.

Chapter 3

McCully K. "The Cholesterol Myth." *The Heart Revolution,* Harper Collins, 1999; 4: 13-17

McCully K. "Why The Low-Cholesterol, Low-Fat Diet Isn't Working." *The Heart Revolution,* Harper Collins 1999; 2:31-48.

Zaret b, Moser M, Cohen I. "The Role Of Cholesterol." *Yale University Heart Book,* Hearst Books 1992, 4: 37-42.

Grahm IM, Daly LE, Refsum HM. "Plasma Homocysteine As A Risk Factor For Vascular Disease." *JAMA* 1997; 277: 1775-1781.

Stuhlinger MC. "Homocysteine Impairs the NO Synthase Pathway— Role Of ADMA." *Circulation* 2001; 104(21): 2569-2575.

Stacey M. "The Rise And Fall Of Kilmer McCully." *New York Times Magazine* 1997.

Sinatra S. "C-Reactive Protein Levels Can Help Predict Heart Disease." *HeartSense,* Nov 2000, P. 6-7.

Sinatra S. "Lp (a) Levels Can Help Predict Future Heart Disease." *HeartSense,* Dec 2000, P. 2-3.

McCully K. "What Is Homocysteine?" *The Heart Revolution,* Harper Collins, 1999; 1:1-27.

Sinatra S. "Homocysteine Levels Can Help Predict Future Heart Disease." *The Sinatra Health Report,* Mar 2001, P. 7-8.

Pirisi A. "How Folic Acid and B Vitamins Reduce Homocysteine." *Life Extension,* Aug 2001; P. 47-52.

Sinatra S. "Coronary Calcification And Fibrinogen." *The Sinatra Health Report,* Feb 2001, P. 6-7.

Chapter 4

Cockcroft J, Wilkinson I. "Arterial Stiffness and Pulse Contour Analysis: An Age Old Concept." *Clincial Science* 2002, 103, 379-380

Hlimoneco I, Meigas K, Vahisalu R. "Waveform Analysis of Peripheral Pulse Wave Detected In The Fingertip With Photoplethysmograph." *Measurement Science Review* 2003, Vol 3, Sec 2, 49-52

Raggi P. "The Use Of Electron-Beam Computed Tomography As A Tool For Primary Prevention." *Am J Cardiol,* 2001, 88(7B): 28J-32J

Forrestor JS. "Prevention Of Plaque Rupture: A New Paradigm Of Therapy." *Ann Int Med,* 137(10): 823-833.

Wayhs R. "High Coronary Artery Calcium Scores Pose An Extremely Elevated Risk For Hard Events." *J Am Coll Cardiol* 2002, 39(2): 225-230

Greenland P, Abrams J. "Beyond Secondary Prevention; Identifying The High-Risk Patient For Primary Prevention; Noninvasive Tests Of Atherosclerosis Burden." *Circulation* 2000, 101:E16-22.

Debaberata M, Yadav J. "Carotid Artery Intimal-Medial Thickness; Indicator Of Atherosclerotic Burden And Response To Risk Factor Modification." *Am Heart J* 2002, 144:753-759

Curtis B, O'Keefe J. "Autonomic Tone As A Cardiovascular Risk Factor." *Mayo Clinic Proc* 2002, 77: 45-54

Chapter 5

Faloon W. "Cardiac Drugs That Cause Heart Attacks." *Life Extension,* June 2003, P. 11-17

Whitaker J. "Cholesterol Drugs: Only As A Last Resort." *Health and Healing,* Jul 2001, P. 1-3.

Whitaker J. "A Cholesterol Lowering Drug Goes Under." *Health and Healing,* Oct 2001, P. 1-3.

Williams D. "Statin Drugs: Risky Business." *Alternatives,* Jan 2002, P. 52-54.

Zarrett B, Moser M, Cohen I. "Cholesterol, Risk, and Common Sense." *Yale University Heart Book,* Hearst Books 1992; 4: 48-49.

Whitaker J. "A Smart Reason To Avoid Bypass Surgery." *Health and Healing,* Apr 2001, P. 1-4.

Whitaker J. "How to Bypass Bypass Surgery." *Health and Healing,* Feb 2002, P. 6-8.

Sinatra S. "Crisis Cardiology." *HeartSense,* Jan 2001; P 6-8

CASS Principal Investigators and the Associates. "Myocardial Infarction and Mortality in the Coronary Artery Bypass Surgery Randomized Trial." *New England Journal of Medicine* 1984; 310: 750-758.

Parisi A, Folland E, Hartigan P. "Comparisons of Angioplasty With Medical Therapy." *New England Journal of Medicine* 1992, *326: 10-16.*

Chapter 6

Castleman M. "Score A Victory Through Vegetarianism." *Blended Medicine,* Rodale 2000; P 334-335.

Cuevas AM. "A High-Fat Diet Induces and Red Wine Counteracts Endothelial Dysfunction In Human Volunteers." *Lipids* 2000; 35(2):143-148.

Vogel RA, Corretti MC, Plotnick GD. The Postprandial Effect Of Components of the Mediterranean Diet On Endothelial Function." *J Am Col Cardiol 2000;* 36(5): 1455-1460.

Zaret B, Moser M, Cohen L. "Adopting A Healthful Diet." *Yale University Heart Book,* Hearst 1992; 5: 51-70.

Frohlich F, Subak-Sharpe G. "Exercise and Your Heart." *Take Heart,* Crown 1990; 8: 133-144.

Hambrecht R. "Regular Exercise Corrects Endothelial Dysfunction and Improves Exercise Capacity In Patients With Chronic Heart Failure." *Circulation* 1998; 98(24): 2709-2715.

Zaret B, Moser M, Cohen l. "The Exercise Prescription." *Yale University Heart Book,* Hearst 1992; 7: 85-94.

Blair SN, Kohl HW, Paffenbarger RS. "Physical Fitness and All-Cause Mortality. A Prospective Study of Men and Women. *JAMA* 1989; 262:2395-2401.

Gielen S, Schuler G, Hambrecht R. "Exercise Training In Coronary Artery Disease and Coronary Vasomotion." *Circulation* 2001; 103: E1-E6.

Hornig B, Maier V, Dresler H. "Physical Training Improves Endothelial Function In Patients With Chronic Heart Failure." *Circulation* 1996; 93:210-214.

Tucker LA, Freidman GM. "Walking and Serum Cholesterol In Adults." *Am J Public Health* 1990; 80:1111-1113.

Fried R, Merrell W. *The Arginine Solution* 1999.

Cooke, J. *The Cardiovascular Cure* 2004.

Ignarro, L. *NO More Heart Disease and Stroke 2005.*

Coffee, C J: Metabolism. Madison, Ct: *Fence Creek Publishing,* 1998; pp: 388-389.

Catt KJ: Molecular Mechanisms of Hormone Action. In Endocrinology and Metabolism, 3rd ed. Edited by Felig P, Baxter JD, Frohman LA. New York, NY: *McGraw-Hill,* 1995, pp 138-139.

Gerhard M, et al. Aging progressively impairs endothelium-dependent vasodilation in forearm resistance vessels of humans. *Hypertension* 1996 Apr;27(4):849-53

Toprakci M, et al. Age-associated changes in nitric oxide metabolites, nitrite and nitrate. *Int J Clin Lab Res* 2000;30(2):83-5

Sakuma I, et al. Identification of arginine as a precursor of endothelium-derived relaxing factor. *Proc Natl Acad Sci USA* 1988 Nov;85(22): 8664-7

Vallance P, Moncada S. Nitric Oxide—from mediator to medicines. *J R Coll Physicians Lond* 1994 May-Jun;28 (3): 209-219

Kam PC, Govender G. Nitric oxide: basic science and clinical applications. *Anaesthesia* 1994 Jun;49(6): 515-21

Sinha G. Viagra: ups and downs. *Popular Science* 2000 July: page 35

Boger RH, Bode-Boger SM, Kienke S, et al. Dietary L-arginine decreases myointimal cell proliferation and vascular monocyte accumulation in cholesterol-fed rabbits. *Atherosclerosis* 1998 Jan;136(1) 67-77

Cheng JW, Balwin SN. L-Arginine in the management of cardiovascular diseases. *Ann Pharmacother* 2001 Jun;35(6):755-64

Tentolouris C, Tousoulis D, et al. L-Arginine in coronary atherosclerosis. *Int J Cardiol* 2000 Sep 15;75(2-3):123-8

Wang B, Ho HV, et al. Regression of atherosclerosis. *Circulation* 1999;99(9):1236-41

Boger RH, Bode-Boger SM, et al. Dietary L-arginine reduces the progression of atherosclerosis in cholesterol fed rabbits: comparison with lovastatin. *Circulation* 1997; 96(4):1282-90

Schuschke DA, Miller FN, Lominadze DG, Feldhoff RC. L-arginine restores cholesterol-attenuated micro vascular responses in the rat cremaster. *Int J Micricirc Clin Exp* 1994 Jul-Aug;14(4): 204-11

Siani A, Pagano E, Iacone R. "Blood Pressure and Metabolic Changes During Dietary L-arginine Supplementation in Humans." *Am J Hypertens* 2000; 13(5 Pt 1): 547-551

Orlandi A, Marcellini M Spagnoli LG. Aging influences development and progression of earl aortic atherosclerosis lesions in cholesterol-fed rabbits. *Arterioscler Thromb Vasac Biol* 2000 Apr;20

Chong PH, Bachenheimer BS. Current, New and future treatments in dyslipidemia and atherosclerosis. *Drugs* 2000 Jul;60(1):55-93

Phivthong-ngam L, Bode-Boger SM, Boger RH, et al. Dietary L-arginine normalizes endothelial induced vascular contractions in cholesterol-fed rabbits. *J Cardiovasc Pharmacol* 1998 Aug;32(2): 300-7

Maxwell AJ, Anderson B Zapien MP, Cooke JP. Endothelial dysfunction in hypercholesterolemia is reversed by: nutritional product designed to enhance nitric oxide activity. *Cardiovasc Drugs Ther* 2000 Jun;14(3): 309-16

Clarkson P, Adams MR, Powe AJ, et al. Oral L-arginine improves endothelial-dependent dilation in hypercholesterolemic young adults. *J Clin Invest* 1996 April; 97(8): 1989-94

Cooke JP, Dzau J, Creager A. Endothelial dysfunction in hypercholesterolemia is corrected by L-arginine. *Basic Res Cardiol* 1991; 86 Suppl 2: 173-81

Fraser GE. Diet and coronary heart disease: beyond dietary fats and low-density-lipoprotein cholesterol. Am J Clin Nutr 1994 May;59(5 Suppl) 1117s-1142sand atherosclerosis. *Drugs* 2000 Jul;60(1):55-93

Quyyumi AA. Does acute improvement of endothelial dysfunction in coronary artery disease improve myocardial ischemia? *J Am Coll Cardiol* 1998 Oct;32(4):904-11

Lerman A, Burnett JC Jr, Higano ST, et al. Long-term L-arginine supplementation improves small vessel coronary endothelial function in humans. *Circulation* 1998 Jun 2;97(21):1648-9

Ceremuzynski L, Chamiec T, Herbaczynska-Cedro K. Effect of supplemental oral L-arginine on exercise capacity in patients with stable angina pectoris. *Am J Cardiol* 1997 Aug 1; 80(3):331-3

Desrois M, Sciaky M, Lan C, et al. L-arginine during long-term ischemia: effects on cardiac function, energetic metabolism and endothelial damage. *J Heart Lung Transplant* 2000 April; 19(4): 367-76

Quyyumi AA, Dakak N, Dodati JG, et al. Effect of L-arginine on human coronary endothelium-dependent and physiologic vasodilation, *J AM Coll Cardiol* 1997 Nov 1; 30(5):1220-7

Egashira K, et al. Effects of L-arginine supplementation on endothelium-dependent coronary vasodilation in patients with angina pectoris and normal coronary arteriograms. *Circulation* 1996;94(2):130-4

Tentoluris C, et al. L-arginine in coronary atherosclerosis. *Int J Cardiol* 2000 Sep15;75(2-3):123-8

Tretjakovs P, Kalnins U, Dabina I, et al. Plasma HDL-cholesterol has an effect on nitric oxide production and arachidonic production in the platelet membranes of coronary artery disease patients without LDL-hypercholesterolemia. *Med Sci Monitor* 2000 May- Jun;6(3):507-11

Bode-Boger SM, Boger RH, Galland A, Tsikas D Frolich JC. L-arginine induced vasodilatation in healthy humans: pharmacokinetic-pharmacodynamic relationship. *Br J Clin Pharmacol* 1998 Nov; 46(5): 489-97

Khedara A, Kawai Y Kayashita J Kato N. Feeding rats the nitric oxide synthase inhibitor, L-N(omega) nitroarginine, elevates serum triglycerides and cholesterol and lowers hepatic fatty acid oxidation. *J Nutr* 1996 Oct;126(10):2563-7

Boger RH, Bode-Boger SM, Theil W, et al. Restoring vascular nitric oxide formation by L-arginine improves symptoms of intermittent claudication in patients with Peripheral arterial occlusive disease. *J Am Col Cardiol* 1998 Nov;32(5):1336-44

Maxwell AJ, Anderson BE Cooke JP. Nutritional therapy for peripheral artery disease. *Vasc Med* 2000;5(1):11-19

Hiatt WR. New treatment options in intermittent claudication: the US experience. *Int J Clin Pract Suppl* 2001 Apr;(119):20-27

Creager MA. Medical management of peripheral artery disease. *Cardiol Rev* 2001 Jul-Aug;9(4):238-45

Korting GE, Smith SD, Wheeler MA, Weiss RM, Foster HE. A randomized double-blind study of oral L-arginine for treatment of interstitial cystitis. *J Urol* 1999 Feb; 161(2):558-65

Cartledge JJ, Davies AM, Eardley I. A randomized double-blind placebo-controlled crossover trial of the efficacy of L-arginine in the treatment of interstitial cystitis. *BJU Int* 2000 Mar; 85(4):421-6

Sisic D, Francishetti A, Frolich ED. Prolonged L-arginine on cardiovascular mass and myocardial hemodynamics and collagen in aged spontaneously hypertensive and normal rats. *Hypertension* 1999 Jan;33(1 Pt 2):451-5

Higashi Y, et al. Effects of L-arginine infusion on renal hemodynamics in patients with mild hypertension. *Hypertension* 1995;25(4):898-902

Hishikawa K, et al. Role of L-arginine-nitric oxide pathway in hypertension. *J Hypertens* 1993 Jun; 11(6):639-45

Dominiczak AF, Bohr DF. Nitric oxide and its' putative role in hypertension. *Hypertension* 1995;25(6):1202-11

Nakaki T, et al. L-arginine induced hypotension. *Lancet* 1990Oct 20; 336(8721):1016-7

Braga M, Gianotti L Raedelli G, et al. Perioperative immunonutrition in patients undergoing cancer surgery: results of a randomized double-blind phase 3 trial. *Arch Surg* 1999 Apr;134(4):428-33

Ghigo E, Aimaretti G, Cornelli G, et al. Diagnosis of GH deficiency in adults. *Growth Hormone IGF Res* 1998 Feb;8 Suppl A:55-8

Wideman L Weltman JY, Patrie JY, et al. Synergy of L-arginine and GHRP-2 stimulation of growth hormone in men and women: modulation by exercise. *Am J Physiol Regul Integr Comp Physiol* 2000 Oct;279(4):R1467-77

Gianotti L, Macario M, Lanfranco F, et al. Arginine counteracts the inhibitory effect of recombinant human insulin-like growth factor I on the somatotroph responsiveness to growth hormone-releasing hormone in humans. *J Clin Endocrinol Metab* 2000 Oct;85(10):3604-8

Mauras N, Walton P, Nicar M, et al. Growth hormone stimulation testing in both short and normal statured children. *Pediatr Res* 2000 Nov;48(5):579-80

Ghigo E, Arvat E, Gianotti L, et al. Hypothalamic growth hormone-insulin-like growth facto-1 axis across the human life span. *J Pediatr Endocrinol Metab* 2000;13 Suppl 6:1493-502

Korbonits M, Kaltsas G, Perry LA, et al. The growth hormone secretagogue hexarelin stimulates the hypothalamo-pituitary-adrenal axis via arginine vasopressin. *J Clin Endocrinol Metab* 1999 Jul;84(7):2489-95

Wallace AW, Ratcliffe MB, Galindez D, Kong JS. L-arginine infusion dilates coronary vasculature in patients undergoing coronary bypass surgery *Aenesthesiology* 1999 Jun;90(6):1577-8

Chen J, Wollman Y, Chernichovsky T, et al. Effect of high dose nitric oxide donor L-arginine in men with organic erectile dysfunction. *BJU Int* 1999 Feb;83(3):269-73

Kobayashi N, Nakamura M, Hiramori K. Effects of infusion of L-arginine on exercise-induced myocardial ischemic changes and capacity to exercise of patients with stable angina pectoris. *Coron Artery Dis* 1999 Jul;10(5):321-6

Bednarz B, Wolk R, Chamiec T, et al. Effects of oral L-arginine supplementation on exercised induced QT dispersion and exercise tolerance in stable angina pectoris. *Int J Cardiol* 2000 Sep 15; 75(2-3). 205-10

De Nicola L, Bellizzi V, Minutolo R, et al. Randomized, double-blind, placebo controlled study of arginine supplementation in chronic renal failure. *Kidney Int* 1999 Aug;56(2):674-84

Watanabe G, Tomiyama H, Doba N. Effects of oral L-arginine on renal function in patients with heart failure. *J Hypertens* 2000 Feb;18(2): 229-34

Kelly BS, Alexander JW Dreyer D, et al. Oral arginine improves blood pressure in renal transplant and hemodialysis patients. *J Parenter Enteral Nutr* 2001 Jul-Aug; 25(4): 194-202

Efron DT, Barbul A. Arginine and nutrition in renal disease. *J Ren Nutr* 1999 Jul;9(3):142-4

Reckelhoff JF, et al. Long-term dietary supplementation with L-arginine prevents age related reduction in renal function. *Am J Physiol* 1997 Jun; 272(6 Pt 2):1768-74

Reyes AA, Purkerson ML, Karl L, Klahr S. Dietary supplementation with L-arginine ameliorates the progression of renal disease in rats with subtotal nephrectomy. *Am J Kidney Dis* 1992 Aug; 20(2):454-5

Bradley SJ, Kingwell BA, McConell GK. Nitric oxide synthase inhibition reduces leg glucose uptake but not blood flow during dynamic exercise in humans. *Diabetes* 1999 Sep; 48(9):1815-21

De Gouw HW, Verbruggen MB, Twiss IM, Sterk PJ. Effect of oral L-arginine on airway hyper-responsiveness to histamine in asthma. *Thorax* 1999 Nov;54(11):1033-5

De Gouw HW, Marshall-Partridge SJ, et al. Role of nitric oxide in the airway response to exercise in healthy and asthmatic subjects. *J Appl Physiol* 2001 Feb;90(2):586-92

Boer J, et al. Role of L-arginine deficiency of nitric oxide and airway hyperreactivity after allergen-induced early asthmatic reaction in guinea-pigs. *Br J Pharmacol* 1999 Nov;128(5):1114-20

Blease K, Kunkel SL, Hogaboam CM. Acute inhibition of nitric oxide exacerbates airway hyperresponsiveness, eosinophilia and C-C chemokine generation in a murinemodel of fungal asthma. *Inflamm Res* 2000 Jun; 49(6):297-304

Gionotti L, Braga M, Fortis C, et al. A prospective, randomized clinical trial on perioperative feeding with an arginine-, omega-3 fatty acid-, and RNA enriched enteral diet: effect on host response and nutritional status. *J Parenter Enteral Nutr* 1999 Nov- Dec;23(6):314-20

Efron D, Barbul A. Role of arginine in immunonutrition. *J Gastroentol* 2000;35 Suppl 12:20-3

Lewis B, Langkamp-Henken B. Arginine enhances in vivo immune responses in young, adult and aged mice. *J Nutri* 2000;130(7):1827-30

Mannick JB, et al. Nitric oxide produced by human B lymphocytes inhibits apoptosis and Epstein-Barr virus reactivation. *Cell* 1994 Dec 30;79(7):1137-46

Ochoa JB, et al. Effects of L-arginine on the proliferation of T-lymphocyte subpopulations. *J Parenter Enteral Nutr* 2001 Jan-Feb;25(1):23-9

di Luigi L, Guidetti L, Pigozzi F, et al. Acute amino acid supplementation enhances pituitary responsiveness in athletes. *Med Sci Sports Exerc* 1999 Dec;31(12):1748-54

Lawecki J et al. Serum insulin, pancreatic glucagons and growth hormone levels in response to intravenous infusion of L-arginine in patients with recently detected juvenile diabetes. *Pol Med Sci Hist Bull* 1976 Apr-Jun;15(2):177-82

Valcenti S, et al Biphasic effect of nitric oxide on testosterone and cyclic GMP productionby purified rat Leydig cells cultured in vivo. *Int J Androl* 1999 Oct; 22(5):336-41

Stevens BR, Godfrey MD, Kaminski TW, Braith RW. High intensity dynamic human muscle performance enhanced by a metabolic intervention. *Med Sci Sports Exerc* 2000 Dec;32(12):2102-8

Piatti PM, Monti LD, Valsecchi G, et al. Long term oral L-arginine administration improves peripheral and hepatic insulin sensitivity in type 2 diabetes. *Diabetes Care* 2001 MAY;24(5):875-80

Giugliana D, et al. Vascular effects of acute hyperglycemia are reversed by L-arginine. *Circulation* 1997; 95(7):1783-90

Mohan IK, Cas UN. Effects of L-arginine-nitric oxide system on chemical induced diabetes mellitus. *Free Radic Biol Med* 1998 Nov 1;25(7):757-65

Mendez JD, Balderas F. Regulation of hyperglycemia and dyslipidemia by exogenous L-arginine in Diabetic rats. *Biochemie* 2001 May;83(5): 453-8

Kaposzta Z, et al. L-arginine and S-nitroglutathione reduce embolization in Humans. *Circulation* 2001;103(19):2371-75

Bode-Boger SM, Boger RH, et al. Differential inhibition of human platelet aggregation and thromboxane A 2 formation by L-arginine in vivo and in vitro. *Arch Pharmacol* 1998; 357:143-150

Wolf A, et al. Dietary L-arginine supplementation normalizes platelet aggregation in hypercholesterolemic humans. *J Am Coll Cardiol* 1997 Mar 1; 29(3):479

Le Yorneau T, Van Belle E, Corseaux D, et al . Role of nitric oxide in re-stenosis after experimental balloon angioplasty in the hypercholesterolemic rabbit. *J Am CollCardiol* 1999 Mar;33(3):876-82

Janero DR, Ewing JF. Nitric Oxide and Postangioplasty re-stenosis: Pathologicalcorrelates and therapeutic potential. *Free Radic Biol Med* 2000 Dec 15;29(12):1199-221

Severin P, et al. Local intramural delivery of l-arginine enhances nitric oxide generation and inhibits lesion formation after balloon angioplasty. *Circulation* 1997;95(7):1863-9

Thomas S, Ramachandran A, Patra S, et al. Nitric oxide protects the intestine from the damage induced by laparotomy and gut manipulation. *J Surg Res* 2001 Jul;99(1):25-32

Sahin AS, Atalik KE, Gunel E, Dogan N. Nonadrenergic, noncholinergic responses of the human colon smooth muscle and the role of K+channels in these responses.. *Methods Find Exp Clin Pharmacol* 2001 Jan-Feb;23(1):13-7

Fini M, et al. Effect of l-lysine and L-arginine on primary osteoblast cultures from normal and osteopenic rats. *Biomed Pharmacother* 2001 May;55(4):213-21

Aikawa K, Yokota T, et al. Endogenous nitric oxide-mediated relaxation and nitrinergic innervation in the rabbit prostate: the change with aging. *Prostate* 2001 Jun 15;48(1):40-6

Suematsu Y, Ohtsuka T, et al. L-Arginine given after ischemic preconditioning can enhance cardioprotection in isolated rat hearts. *Eur J Cardiothorac Surg* 2001, Jun;19(6):873-9

Koglin J. Pathogenetic mechanisms of cardiac allograft vasculopathy-impact of nitric oxide. *Z Kardiol* 2000;89 Suppl 9:IX/24-7

Kown MH, Van Der Steenhoven T, Uemura S, et al. L-Arginine polymer mediated inhibition of graft coronary artery disease after cardiac transplantation. *Transplantation* 2001 June 15;71(11):1542-8

Freedman RR, Girgis R, Mayers MD. Acute effect if nitric oxide on Raynaud's phenomenon in scleroderma. *Lancet* 1999 Aug 28:354;739

Morric CR, Kuypers FA, et al. Patterns of arginine and nitric oxide in patients with sickle cell disease with vaso-occlusive crisis and acute chest syndrome. *J Ped Hemat/Onc* 2000 Nov-Dec;22(6):515-20

Kumar CA, Das UN. Lipid peroxides, antioxidants and nitric oxide in patients with pre-eclampsia and essential hypertension. *Med Sci Monitor* 2000 Sep-Oct;6(5):901-7

Nagaya N, Uematsu M, et al. Short term oral administration of l-arginine improves hemodynamics and exercise capacity in patients with precapillary pulmonary hypertension. *Am J Resp Crit Care Med* 2001 April;163(4):887-91

Barbul A, et al. Arginine enhances wound healing and lymphocyte immune responsesin humans. *Surgery* 1990 Aug;108(2):331-6; discussion 336-7

Kirk SJ, et al Arginine stimulates wound healing and immune function in elderly humans. *Surgery* 1993 Aug;114(2):155-9; discussion 160

De-Souza DA, Greene LJ. Pharmacological nutrition after burn injury. *J of Nutri* 1998 May;128(5):797-803

Blum A, Cannon RO, Costello R, et al. Endocrine and lipid effects of oral L-arginine treatment in healthy postmenopausal women. *J Lab Clin Med* 2000 Mar;135(3):231-7

Ohta Y, Nishida K., Protective effect of l-arginine against stress-induced gastric mucosal lesions in rats and its relation to nitric acid-mediated inhibition of neutrophil infiltration. *Pharmacal Res* 2001 Jun;43(6):535-41

Khattab MM, Gad MZ, Abdallah D. Protective role of nitric oxide in indomethacin- induced gastric ulceration by a mechanism independent of gastric acid secretion. *Pharmacol Res* 2001 May;43(5):463-7

Calver A, Collier J, Vallance P. Dilator actions of arginine in human peripheral vasculature. *Clin Sci* 1991 Nov;81(5):695-700

Bode-Boger SM, Boger RH,et al. L-arginine induces nitric oxide-dependent vasodilation in patients with critical limb ischemia. A randomized, controlled study. *Circulation* 1996 Jan 1; 93(1):85-90

Vallet B. Microthrombosis in sepsis. *Minerva Anestesiol* 2001 Apr;67(4):298-301.

Hambrecht R, et al. Correction of endothelial dysfunction in chronic heart failure: additional effects of exercise training and oral L-arginine supplementation. *J Am Coll Cardiol* 2000 Mar 1; 35(3):706-13

Heys SD, et al. Dietary supplementation with L-arginine: Modulation of tumor infiltrating lymphocytes in patients with colo-rectal cancer. *Br J Surg* 1997 Feb;84(2):238-41

Brittenden J, et al. Dietary supplementation with L-arginine in patients with breast cancer(> 4cm.) receiving multi-modality treatment: report of a feasibility study. *Br J Cancer* 1994 May;69(5):918-21

McCarty MF. Vascular nitric oxide, sex hormone replacement, and fish oil may help to prevent Alzheimer's disease by suppressing synthesis of acute-phase cytokines. *Med Hypotheses* 1999 Nov;53(3):369-74

Tarkowski E, et al. Intrathecal release of nitric oxide in Alzheimer's disease and vascular dementia. *Dement Geriatr Cogn Disord* 2000 Nov-Dec;11(6):322-6

de la Torre JC, Stefano GB. Evidence that Alzheimer's disease is a microvascular disorder: the role of constitutive nitric oxide. *Brain Res Brain Res Rev* 2000 Dec;34(3):119-36

Kuiper MA, et al. Decrease cerebrospinal fluid nitrate levels in Parkinson's disease, Alzheimer's disease and multiple system atrophy patients. *J Neurol Sci* 1994 Jan; 121(1):46-9

Pautler EL. The possible role and treatment of deficient microcirculation regulation in age-associated memory impairment. *Med Hypotheses* 1994 Jun;42(6):363-6

Pandhi P, Balakrishnan S. Cognitive dysfunction induced by phenytoin and valproate in rats: effect of nitric oxide. *Indian J Physiol Pharmacol* 1999 Jul; 43(3):378-82

Pendergast MA, et al. Nitric oxide synthase inhibition impairs delayed recall in mature monkeys. *Pharmacol Biochem Behav* 1997 Jan;56(1):81-7

Fideieff HL,et al. Reproducibility and safety of the arginine test in normal adults. *Medicina* (B Aires) 1999; 59(3):249-53

Fagan JM, et al. L-arginine reduces right heart hypertrophy in hypoxia-induced pulmonary hypertension. *Biochem Biophys Res Commun* 1999 Jan 8; 254(1):100-3

Nitric oxide and pulmonary hypertension. *Coron Artery Dis* 1999 Jul; 10(5):287-94

Maxwell A, Anderson B, Zapien M, Cooke J. "Endothelial Dysfunction in Hypercholesrolemia." *Cardiovascular Drugs and Therapy* 2000; 14:309-316.

Maxwell A, Cooke J. "L Arginine: Its Role in Cardiovascular Therapy." *Contemporary Cardiology* 2001; 30:1-25.

Maxwell A, Zapien M, Pearce G, MacCallum G, Stone P. "Randomized Trial of a Medical Food for the Dietary Management of Chronic, Stable Angina." *Journal of the American College of Cardiology* Jan 2002; P 37-45.

Sinatra S. "Chelation Therapy: Fact or Fiction." *The Sinatra Health Report,* May 2001, P. 2-5; Jun 2001 P. 3-5.

Harman D. "The Biologic Clock: The Mitochondria?" *Journal of American Geriatrics* 1972; 20:145-147.

Clarke N, Clarke C, Mosher R. "Treatment of Angina Pectoris With Disodium Ethelyne Diamene Tetraacetic Acid." *American Journal of Medical Science* Dec 1956; 654-666.

Hancke C, Flytile K. "Benefits of EDTA Chelation Therapy in Arteriosclerosis." *Journal of Advancement in Medicine* 1993; 6:3, 161-171.

Chappell L, Janson M. "EDTA Chelation Therapy in the Treatment of Vascular Disease." *Journal of Cardiovascular Nurses* 1996; 10:78-86.

Balch J, Balch P. "Elements of Health: Antioxidants." *Prescription for Nutritional Healing,* Avery 1997; P43-46.

Enstrom JE, Kanim LE, Klein MA. "Vitamin C Intake and Mortality Among A Sample of the U.S. Population. *Epidemiology* 1992; 3:194-202.

Rimm EB, Stampfer MJ, Ascherio A. "Vitamin E Consumption and the Risk Of Coronary Artery Disease In Men." *N Eng J Med* 1993; 328: 1487-1489.

Schnyder G, Roffi M, Flammer Y. "Effect of Homocysteine-Lowering Therapy With Folic Acid, Vitamin B12 and Vitamin B6 On Clinical Outcome After Percutaneous Coronary Intervention." *JAMA* 2002; 288: 973-979

Langsjoen H, Langsjoen P. "Usefulness of Coenzyme Q-10 In Clinical Cardiology: A Long Term Study." *Mol Aspects Med* 1994; 15 Suppl: S165-175.

Friedrich MJ. "To E Or Not To E, Vitamin E's role In Health and Disease Is the Question." *JAMA* 2004; 292: 671-673.

Fetrow C, Avila J. "Tumeric." The Complete Guide to Herbal Medicines, *Springhouse* 2000; P. 494-495.

Null G. "Heart Disease: Supplements." *Natural Healing,* Kensington 2001; P. 208-212.

Maleskey G. "Heart Disease: Supplements." *Nature's Medicine,* Rodale 1999; P. 464-484.

Gottlieb B. "Natural Remedies To Stop Heart Disease." *Alternative Cures* Rodale 2000; P. 332-334.

Castleman M. "Curing Yourself of Heart Disease." *Blended Medicine,* Rodale 2000; P. 342-344.

White L, Foster S. "Vitamins For Heart Health." *The Herbal Drugstore,* Rodale 2000; P. 304-308.

Pirisi A. "How Folic Acid and B Vitamins Reduce Homocysteine." *Life Extension,* Aug 2001; P. 47-52.

Prevention. "Heart Disease: Low Levels of Nutrients Put You At Risk." *Healing With Vitamins,* Rodale 1996, P. 288-296.

Chambers JC. "Demonstration of Rapid Onset Vascular Endothelial Dysfunction After Hyperhomocysteinemia: An Effect Reversible By Vitamin C Therapy." *Circulation* 1999; 99: 1156-1160.

Taddei S. "Vitamin C Improves Endothelium-Dependent Vasodilation By Restoring Nitric Oxide Activity In Essential Hypertension." *Circulation* 1998; 97: 2222-2229.

Kris-Etherton PM, Etherton TD, Yu S. "Efficacy of Multiple Dietary Therapies In Reducing Cardiovascualr Risk Factors." *Am J Clin Nutr* 1997; 65: 560.

Balch J., Balch P. "Supplements For Cardiovascular Disease." *Prescription for Nutritional Healing,* Avery 1997; P. 187-190.

Sinatra S. "CoQ10 Works. Period." *The Sinatra Health Report,* Feb 2001, P. 3-5.

Whitaker J. "A Hormone That Can Help." *Reverse Your Heart Disease Naturally,* Phillips 1999; P. 16-17.

Whitaker J. "Targeted Supplementation." *Reverse Your Heart Disease Naturally,* Phillips 1999; P. 11-12.

Diplock AT. "Antioxidant Nutrients and Disease Prevention: An Overview." *Amer J Clin Nutrit* 1991; 53(1 Suppl): 189S-193S

Cacciatore L. "The Therapeutic Effect of L-Carnitine In Patients Exercise-Induced Stable Angina: A Controlled Study." *Drugs Exp Clin Res* 1991; 17(4): 225-235.

Davini P. "Controlled Study On L-Carnitine therapeutic Efficacy In Post-Infarction." *Drugs Exp Clin Res* 1992; 18(8): 355-365.

Hofman-Bang C. "Coenzyme Q10 As An Adjunctive Treatment of Congestive Heart Failure." *J Am Coll Cardiol* 1992 19: 216A.

Mortenson SA. "Coenzyme Q10: Clinical Benefits With Biochemical Correlates Suggesting A Scientific Breakthrough in the Management of Chronic Heart Failure." *Int J Tissue React* 1990; 12(3): 155-162.

Weber C. "Antioxidant Effect of Dietary Coenzyme Q10 in Human Blood Plasma." *Int J Vitam Nutr Res* 1994; 64(4): 311-315.

Whitaker J. "Fish Oil and Heart Disease." *Health and Healing,* Nov 2000; P.5.

Albert C, Camos H, Manson J. "Blood Levels of Long-Chain n-3 Fatty Acids and the Rish of Sudden Death." *New England Journal of Medicine* 2002, Vol 346: 1113-1118.

Sacks EM. "Controlled Trial of Fish Oils For Regression of Human Coronary Atherosclereosis." *J Am col Cardiol* 1995; 25: 1492-1498.

De Lorgeril M. "Mediterranean Alpha-Linolenic Acid-Rich Diet In Secondary Prevention of Coronary Heart disease." *Lancet* 1994; 343: 1454-1459.

Adler AJ. "Effect of Garlic and Fish Oil Supplementation On Serum Lipid and Liporotein Concentrations In Hypercholesterolemic Men." *Am J Clin Nutr* 1997; 65: 445-460.

Whitaker J. "Nature's Miracle Drug." *Reverse Your Heart Disease Naturally,* Phillips 1999, P: 15-16.

Auguet M. "Ginkgo Biloba Extract and the Regulation of Vascular Tone." *Advances in ginkgo Biloba Extract Research* 1994; (Egb 761).

Chang WC. "Inhibition of Platelet Aggregation and Arachidonate Metabolism in Platelets By Procyanidins." *Prostaglandins Leukot Essent Fatty Acids* 1989; 38: 181-188.

Frankel EN. "Inhibition of Oxidation of Human Low-Density Lipoprotein By Phenolic Substances In Red Wine." *Lancet* 1993; 341: 454-457.

Hertog MG. "Dietary Antioxidant Flavonoids and Risk of Coronary Heart disease>" *Lancet* 1993; 342: 1007-1111.

Neve J. "Selenium As A Risk Factor For Cardiovascular Disease." *J Cardiovasc Risk* 1996; 3(1): 42-47.

Whitaker J. "EECP vs Bypass Surgery." *Reverse Your Heart Disease Naturally,* Phillips 1999, P. 17-18.

Sinatra S. "Putting The Squeeze On Heart Disease." *The Sinatra Health Report,* Feb 2001, P. 7-8.

Ubbink J, Vermaak W, Vander M. "Vitamin Requirements For The Treatment Of Hyperhomocysteinemia In Humans." *Journal of Nutrition* 1994, 124:1927-1983.

Family Nutrition "Policosanol Lowers Cholestero.l" *Gynecological Endocrinology,* 14(3): 187-95, 2000, Angiology 2001, 52(2):115-25.

ABOUT THE AUTHOR

Harry Elwardt is a Naturopathic Doctor, Master Herbalist and Certified Nutritional Counselor. He is also the CEO and Founder of *The Health Guardian*™, a website and workshop program dedicated to the education of holistic healing. He has received his diplomas from *The Trinity College Of Natural Health* located in Warsaw, Indiana. He also has earned a Ph.D. in Health & Nutrition from the prestigious *University of Hampshire* located in London, England. He has been working in the alternative medicine field for 10 years and is passionate about helping people through naturopathic therapies. He has been a featured speaker on many radio and television programs. He also serves on the Medical Advisory Board for *ArkWorld International, ForMor International, Life Mission International and Nutrition & Kids*.

Dr. Harry believes the real cause for disease and death is medical ignorance and through personal education and a good, strategic nutritional supplement program, wellness can be achieved. Dr. Harry has formulated cutting edge nutraceuticals for several companies.

Dr. Harry is taking his message of hope to organizations, churches, schools, health food stores, and fitness centers across America. He is offering an explosive seminar with an eye opening PowerPoint presentation that will change the lives of everyone who attends. To make arrangements for Dr. Harry to a workshop at your location and/or a Digital Pulsewave cardiovascular screening, please call **(630) 961-5145** or e-mail Dr. Harry at drharry@wideopenwest.com or visit Dr. Harry's website at **www.thehealthguardian.com.**

"It's time to *"Wake Up America"* and take affirmative action in restoring wellness throughout our great country!"

Dr. Harry resides in Naperville, Illinois with his wife of 29 years, Cathy, and his 3 children Dana, Lindsay and Jonathan.